Practice Test #1

Practice Questions

Verbal Review

1. Jerry held out hope for recovery, in spite of the *ominous* results from the lab.
Ominous means:
    a. threatening
    b. emboldening
    c. destructive
    d. insightful

2. The *occluded* artery posed a significant threat to the long-term health of the patient.
Occluded means:
    a. closed
    b. deformed
    c. enlarged
    d. engorged

3. The doctors were less concerned with Bill's respiration than with the *precipitous* rise in his blood pressure.
Precipitous means:
    a. detached
    b. sordid
    c. encompassed
    d. steep

4. It is *vital* for the victim of a serious accident to receive medical attention immediately.
Vital means:
    a. recommended
    b. discouraged
    c. essential
    d. sufficient

5. Wracked by abdominal pain, the victim of food poisoning moaned and rubbed his *distended* belly.
Distended means:
    a. concave
    b. sore
    c. swollen
    d. empty

60.73069
P341
2014
c.2

6. Despite the absence of *overt* signs, Dr. Harris suspected that Alicia might be suffering from the flu.
Overt means:
  a. concealed
  b. apparent
  c. expert
  d. delectable

7. The medication should only be taken if the old symptoms *recur*.
Recur means:
  a. occur again
  b. survive
  c. collect
  d. desist

8. At first, Gerald suspected that he had caught the disease at the office; later, though, he concluded that it was *endogenous.*
Endogenous means:
  a. contagious
  b. painful to the touch
  c. continuous
  d. growing from within

9. Though chemotherapy had sent her cancer into remission, Glenda remained *lethargic* and depressed.
Lethargic means:
  a. nauseous
  b. sluggish
  c. contagious
  d. elated

10. In order to minimize scarring, the nurse reused the *site* of the previous injection.
Site means:
  a. syringe
  b. location
  c. artery
  d. hole

11. As a veteran of many flu seasons, the nurse knew how to minimize her *exposure* to the disease.
Exposure means:
  a. laying open
  b. prohibition
  c. connection
  d. dislike

12. Dr. Grant ignored Mary's particular symptoms, instead administering a *holistic* treatment for her condition.
Holistic means:
    a. insensitive
    b. ignorant
    c. specialized
    d. concerned with the whole rather than the parts

13. The dermatologist was struck by the *symmetric* patterns of scarring on the patient's back.
Symmetric means:
    a. scabbed
    b. painful to the touch
    c. occurring in corresponding parts at the same time
    d. geometric

14. Despite an increase in the *volume* of his urine, the patient still reported bloating.
Volume means:
    a. quality
    b. length
    c. quantity
    d. loudness

15. The group hiked along a *precipitous* slope that many found unnerving.
Precipitous means:
    a. rugged
    b. dangerous
    c. steep
    d. wet

16. Saline is taking a philosophy class but finds most of the readings to be very *obscure*, so she has not benefited much from them.
Obscure means:
    a. opinionated
    b. unclear
    c. offensive
    d. benign

17. As a young boy, Dorian was *remiss* about his homework and failed to get good grades in school.
Remiss means:
    a. timely
    b. diligent
    c. negligent
    d. meticulous

18. In the movie, the lead actress thought the lead actor was a burglar and *brandished* a stick at him in a threatening manner.
Brandished means:
    a. threw
    b. waved menacingly
    c. smacked
    d. peered

19. Stanley was so *besotted* with his prom date that he spent most of the dance gazing at her adoringly.
Besotted means:
    a. infatuated
    b. infuriated
    c. perplexed
    d. engrossed

20. Since he was in the *vicinity* of his mom's house, he decided to drop by and see if she was home.
Vicinity means:
    a. neighborhood
    b. parish
    c. mindset
    d. idea

21. After practice, the girl's softball team stated, "We're *famished*!"
Famished means
    a. Fatigued
    b. Hungry
    c. Excited
    d. Ready

22. The newborn baby was *enamored* with the rattle.
Enamored means
    a. Fascinated
    b. Happy
    c. Unsure what to do
    d. Aggravated

23. When having a problem, it is best to *dissect* the situation then act.
Dissect means
    a. Cut apart
    b. Talk about
    c. Ignore
    d. Analyze

24. The child *apprized* her father's authority and behaved herself in church.
Apprized means
    a. Appreciated
    b. Compromised
    c. Defied
    d. Noted

25. John's chart notes that he has *pallid* skin.
Pallid means:
    a. sallow
    b. pale
    c. sanguine
    d. sickly

26. Marie's chart indicates that she should receive *diurnal* administration of an antibiotic.
Diurnal means:
    a. continuous
    b. nightly
    c. daily
    d. parenteral

27. You become concerned about a patient because they are in a state of *confusion*.
Confusion means:
    a. agitation
    b. certitude
    c. indifference
    d. bewilderment

28. A laboratory report indicates that the patient's blood fails to *coagulate*.
Coagulate means:
    a. clot
    b. deliquesce
    c. solidify
    d. separate

29. After listening to Bob's breathing, the doctor indicates that it is *cadenced*.
Cadenced means:
    a. normal
    b. rhythmic
    c. irregular
    d. regular

30. An *impending* stroke may be indicated by headache, dizziness, double vision, and other deficiencies.
Impending means:
    a. eventual
    b. prophetic
    c. imminent
    d. portentous

31. The doctor's explanation of his diagnosis was too *obscure*.
Obscure means:
    a. confounding
    b. unclear
    c. ambiguous
    d. straightforward

32. The patient strives to act in *compliance* with her parents' wishes.
Compliance means:
    a. complaisance
    b. defiance
    c. acquiescence
    d. deference

33. The patient's chart was *rife* with errors.
Rife means:
    a. devoid
    b. fraught
    c. transcribed
    d. overloaded

34. Anna just has been diagnosed with breast cancer, and she faces a *quandary*.
Quandary means:
    a. impasse
    b. decision
    c. heartbreak
    d. dilemma

35. The insurance company *disavowed* the patient's claim.
Disavowed means:
    a. approved
    b. rejected
    c. disclaimed
    d. acknowledged

Questions 36 – 43 pertain to the following passage:

VISUAL PERCEPTION

It is tempting to think that your eyes are simply mirrors that reflect whatever is in front of them. Researchers, however, have shown that your brain is constantly working to create the impression of a continuous, uninterrupted world.

For instance, in the last ten minutes, you have blinked your eyes around 200 times. You have probably not been aware of any of these interruptions in your visual world. Something you probably have not seen in a long time without the aid of a mirror is your nose. It is always right there, down in the bottom corner of your vision, but your brain filters it out so that you are not aware of your nose unless you purposefully look at it.

Nor are you aware of the artery that runs right down the middle of your retina. It creates a large blind spot in your visual field, but you never notice the hole it leaves. To see this blind spot, try the following: Cover your left eye with your hand. With your right eye, look at the O on the left. As you move your head closer to the O, the X will disappear as it enters the blind spot caused by your optical nerve.

O   X

Your brain works hard to make the world look continuous!

36. The word <u>filters</u>, as used in this passage, most nearly means:
   a. Alternates
   b. Reverses
   c. Ignores
   d. Depends

37. The word <u>retina</u>, as used in this passage, most nearly means:
   a. Optical illusion
   b. Part of the eye
   c. Pattern
   d. Blindness

38. Which of the following statements can be inferred from this passage?
   a. Not all animals' brains filter out information.
   b. Visual perception is not a passive process.
   c. Blind spots cause accidents.
   d. The eyes never reflect reality.

39. What is the author's purpose for including the two letters in the middle of the passage?
   a. To demonstrate the blind spot in the visual field.
   b. To organize the passage.
   c. To transition between the last two paragraphs of the passage.
   d. To prove that the blind spot is not real.

40. What is the main purpose of this passage?
   a. To persuade the reader to pay close attention to blind spots.
   b. To explain the way visual perception works.
   c. To persuade the reader to consult an optometrist if the O and X disappear.
   d. To prove that vision is a passive process.

41. Based on the passage, which of the following statements is true?
   a. The brain cannot accurately reflect reality.
   b. Glasses correct the blind spot caused by the optical nerve.
   c. Vision is the least important sense.
   d. The brain fills in gaps in the visual field.

42. The author mentions the nose to illustrate what point?
   a. The brain filters out some visual information.
   b. Not all senses work the same way.
   c. Perception is a passive process.
   d. The sense of smell filters out information.

43. Which of the following statements can be inferred from the second paragraph?
    a. The brain filters out the sound created by the shape of the ears.
    b. The brain does not perceive all activity in the visual field.
    c. Closing one eye affects depth perception.
    d. The brain evolved as a result of environmental factors.

Questions 44 -51 pertain to the following passage:

OPPOSITIONAL DEFIANT DISORDER

On a bad day, have you ever been irritable? Have you ever used a harsh tone or even been verbally disrespectful to your parents or teachers? Everyone has a short temper from time to time, but current statistics indicate that between 16% and 20% of a school's population suffer from a psychological condition known as Oppositional Defiance Disorder, or ODD.

ODD symptoms include difficulty complying with adult requests, excessive arguments with adults, temper tantrums, difficulty accepting responsibility for actions, low frustration tolerance, and behaviors intended to annoy or upset adults. Parents of children with ODD can often feel as though their whole relationship is based on conflict after conflict.

Unfortunately, ODD can be caused by a number of factors. Some students affected by ODD suffer abuse, neglect, and severe or unpredictable discipline at home. Others have parents with mood disorders or have experienced family violence. Various types of therapy are helpful in treating ODD, and some drugs can treat particular symptoms. However, no single cure exists.

The best advice from professionals is directed toward parents. Therapists encourage parents to avoid situations that usually end in power struggles, to try not to feed into oppositional behavior by reacting emotionally, to praise positive behaviors, and to discourage negative behaviors with timeouts instead of harsh discipline.

44. Which of the following best describes the main idea of this passage?
    a. ODD has no cause.
    b. ODD is a complex condition.
    c. Parents with ODD should seek support.
    d. Parents are the cause of ODD.

45. As used in this passage, the word oppositional most nearly means:
    a. Uncooperative
    b. Violent
    c. Passive aggressive
    d. Altruistic

46. Which of the following can be inferred from paragraph one?
    a. Most children who speak harshly to their parents have ODD.
    b. Most people exhibit symptoms of ODD occasionally.
    c. Between 16% and 20% of the school population has been abused.
    d. A short temper is a symptom of obsessive compulsive disorder.

47. As used in this passage, the phrase <u>feed into</u> most nearly means:
    a. Discourage
    b. Ignore
    c. Encourage
    d. Abuse

48. As used in this passage, the phrase <u>low frustration tolerance</u> most nearly means:
    a. Patience
    b. Low IQ
    c. Difficulty dealing with frustration
    d. The ability to cope with frustration

49. The author's purpose in writing this passage is to:
    a. Express frustration about ODD.
    b. Prove that parents are the cause of ODD.
    c. Inform the reader about this complex condition.
    d. Persuade the reader to keep students with ODD out of public school.

50. According to the passage, which of the following is a cause of ODD?
    a. Excessive television viewing.
    b. Poor diet.
    c. Severe or unpredictable punishment.
    d. Low IQ.

51. Based on the passage, which of the following statements seems most true?
    a. A variety of parenting techniques can be used to help children with ODD.
    b. Children with ODD must be physically aggressive to be diagnosed.
    c. Parents of children with ODD often engage in risk-taking activities.
    d. Harsh disciplinary measures must be used to control children with ODD.

Questions 52 – 55 pertain to the following passage:

Protozoa are microscopic, one-celled organisms that can be free-living or parasitic in nature. They are able to multiply in humans, a factor which contributes to their survival and also permits serious infections to develop from just a single organism. Transmission of protozoa that live in the human intestine to another human typically occurs by a fecal-oral route (for example, contaminated food or water, or person-to-person contact). Protozoa that thrive in the blood or tissue of humans are transmitted to their human hosts by an arthropod vector (for example, through the bite of a mosquito or sand fly).

Helminths are large, multicellular organisms that are generally visible to the naked eye in their adult stages. Like protozoa, helminths can be either free-living or parasitic in nature. In their adult form, helminths cannot multiply in humans. There are three main groups of helminths (derived from the Greek word for worms) that are human parasites:

1. Flatworms (platyhelminths) – these include the trematodes (flukes) and cestodes (tapeworms).

- 11 -

2. Thorny-headed worms (acanthocephalins) – the adult forms of these worms reside in the gastrointestinal tract. The acanthocephala are thought to be intermediate between the cestodes and nematodes.

3. Roundworms (nematodes) – the adult forms of these worms can reside in the gastrointestinal tract, blood, lymphatic system or subcutaneous tissues. Alternatively, the immature (larval) states can cause disease through their infection of various body tissues.

52. As used in this passage, the word "parasite" means
    a. a person who lives in Paris
    b. an organism that live on or in another organism
    c. microscopic insects
    d. a person who takes advantage of the generosity of others

53. According to the passage, adult Roundworms can live in
    a. the arthropod vector
    b. fecal matter
    c. the subcutaneous tissue of humans
    d. contaminated water

54. You can infer from this passage that
    a. larval stages of parasites are more dangerous than the adult forms
    b. mosquitoes do not transmit parasites
    c. worms cannot infect humans
    d. clean sanitary conditions will keep you free of protozoa

55. According to the passage, which of the following is true?
    I.   Protozoa live in the blood or tissue of humans.
    II.   Adult helminthes cannot reproduce in humans.
    III.   Adult Thorny-headed worms live in the intestinal tract.
    a. I only
    b. II only
    c. I and II only
    d. I, II, and III

Questions 56 – 58 pertain to the following passage:
About 17 million children and adults in the United States suffer from asthma, a condition that makes it hard to breathe. Today it is a problem that is treatable with modern medicine. In days gone by, there were many different superstitions about how to cure asthma. Some people thought that eating crickets with a little wine would help. Eating raw cat's meat might be the cure. Another idea was to try gathering some spiders' webs, rolling them into a ball, and then swallowing them. People also thought that if you ate a diet of only boiled carrots for two weeks, your asthma might go away. This carrot diet may have done some good for asthma patients since vitamin A in carrots is good for the lungs.

56. Which of the following would be a good title for the passage?
    a. Asthma in the United States
    b. Methods of treating asthma
    c. Old wives' tales
    d. Superstitions about asthma

57. The fact that 17 million children and adults in the United States suffer from asthma is probably the opening sentence of the passage because:
    a. It explains why people in times gone by might have found a need to try homemade cures.
    b. It creates a contrast between today and the past.
    c. It lets the reader know that many people have asthma.
    d. It is a warning that anyone could get asthma.

58. The main purpose of the passage is to:
    a. Describe herbal remedies
    b. Explain some of the measures for treating asthma from long ago
    c. Define superstitions
    d. Extol the virtues of modern medicine

Questions 59 – 60 pertain to the following passage:

During the last 100 years of medical science, the drugs that have been developed have altered the way people live all over the world. Over-the-counter and prescription drugs are now the key for dealing with diseases, bodily harm, and medical issues. Drugs like these are used to add longevity and quality to people's lives. But not all drugs are healthy for every person. A drug does not necessarily have to be illegal to be abused or misused. Some ways that drugs are misused include taking more or less of the drug than is needed, using a drug that is meant for another person, taking a drug for longer than needed, taking two or more drugs at a time, or using a drug for a reason that has nothing to do with being healthy. Thousands of people die from drug misuse or abuse every year in the United States.

59. According to the passage, which of the following is an example of misusing a drug?
    a. taking more of a prescription drug than the doctor ordered
    b. taking an antibiotic to kill harmful bacteria
    c. experiencing a side effect from an over-the-counter drug
    d. throwing away a medication that has passed the expiration date

60. According to the passage, which of the following is not true?
    a. over-the-counter drugs are used for medical issues
    b. every year, thousands of people in the United States die due to using drugs the wrong way
    c. medical science has come a long way in the last century
    d. all drugs add longevity to a person's life

Mathematics Review

61.   236
      +301

   a. 505
   b. 507
   c. 535
   d. 537

62.   4,307
      +1,864

   a. 5,161
   b. 5,271
   c. 6,171
   d. 6,271

63. If $a = 3$ and $b = -2$, what is the value of $a^2 + 3ab - b^2$?
   a. 5
   b. -13
   c. -4
   d. -20

64.   356
      -167

   a. 189
   b. 198
   c. 211
   d. 298

65.   5,306
      -3,487

   a. 1,181
   b. 1,819
   c. 2,119
   d. 2,189

66. 34 is what percent of 80?
   a. 34%
   b. 40%
   c. 42.5%
   d. 44.5%

67.   707
   x 17

    a. 12,019
    b. 12,049
    c. 17,019
    d. 17,049

68. $7\overline{)917}$
    a. 131
    b. 131 R4
    c. 145
    d. 145 R4

69. Factor the following expression: $x^2 + x - 12$
    a. $(x - 4)(x + 4)$
    b. $(x - 2)(x + 6)$
    c. $(x + 6)(x - 2)$
    d. $(x + 4)(x - 3)$

70. 38/100 as a decimal
    a. 0.38
    b. 0.038
    c. 3.8
    d. 0.0038

71.   6.8
    11.3
  + 0.06

    a. 17.16
    b. 17.70
    c. 18.16
    d. 18.70

72. The average of six numbers is 4. If the average of two of those numbers is 2, what is the average of the other four numbers?
    a. 5
    b. 6
    c. 7
    d. 8

73. Which numeral is in the thousandths place in 0.3874?
    a. 3
    b. 8
    c. 7
    d. 4

74. 0.58 - 0.39=
    a. 0.19
    b. 1.9
    c. 0.29
    d. 2.9

75. Solve: 0.25 x 0.03 =
    a. 75
    b. 0.075
    c. 0.75
    d. 0.0075

76. 3 1/8 + 6 + 3/7 =
    a. 9 31/56
    b. 9 1/2
    c. 9 21/56
    d. 9 7/8

77. 4 1/7 – 2 1/2 =
    a. 2 5/14
    b. 1 5/14
    c. 1 9/14
    d. 2 9/14

78. 1 1/4 × 3 2/5 × 1 2/3 =
    a. 7 1/12
    b. 5 5/6
    c. 6 7/12
    d. 8 11/15

79. How many 3-inch segments can a 4.5-yard line be divided into?
    a. 15
    b. 45
    c. 54
    d. 64

80. Reduce 14/98 to lowest terms.
    a. 7/49
    b. 2/14
    c. 1/7
    d. 3/8

81. Thirty six hundredths as a percent.
    a. 36%
    b. .36%
    c. .036%
    d. 3.6%

82. 40% of 900
    a. 280
    b. 340
    c. 360
    d. 420

83. Sheila, Janice, and Karen, working together at the same rate, can complete a job in 3 1/3 days. Working at the same rate, how much of the job could Janice and Karen do in one day?
    a. 1/5
    b. 1/4
    c. 1/3
    d. 1/9

84. Three eighths of forty equals:
    a. 15
    b. 20
    c. 22
    d. 24

85. 6% of 25
    a. .3
    b. 1.5
    c. 3.0
    d. 15

86. Ratio of 4 to 16 = (?)%
    a. 2
    b. 4
    c. 12
    d. 25

87. $4^6 \div 2^8$
    a. 2
    b. 8
    c. 16
    d. 32

88. 30% as a reduced common fraction
    a. 30/100
    b. 1/30
    c. 23/10
    d. 3/10

89. 37% as a decimal
    a. .0037
    b. .037
    c. .37
    d. 3.7

90. -4a + 6a + 2a
    a. 4a
    b. -4a
    c. 8a
    d. 12a

91. If $a = 4$, $b = 3$, and $c = 1$, then $\dfrac{a(b-c)}{b(a+b+c)} =$
    a. 4/13
    b. 1/3
    c. 1/4
    d. 1/6

92. $(x^2 - 3x + 3) - (x^2 + 3x - 3)$
    a. 0
    b. $2x^2$
    c. $3x - 3$
    d. $-6x + 6$

93. $4y + 5 = 21$
    a. $y = 3$
    b. $y = 4$
    c. $y = 5$
    d. $y = 6$

94. $3(x + 14) = 4(x + 9)$
    a. $x = 4$
    b. $x = 6$
    c. $x = 12$
    d. $x = 15$

95. What is 20% of 12/5, expressed as a percentage?
    a. 48%
    b. 65%
    c. 72%
    d. 76%

96. A rectangle where the width is 10 feet and the height is 15 feet.
 Which of the following equations is correct for finding the perimeter of the rectangle?
    a. 10 x 15
    b. 10 x 10 x 15 x 15
    c. (10 + 10)(15 + 15)
    d. 2(10) + 2(15)

97. In a graduating high school class of 532, 15% of the students will receive A's and 55% of the students will receive B's. If 53 students receive D's and no one failed, what approximate percentage of the students received C's?

    a. 10%
    b. 20%
    c. 30%
    d. 40%

98. 5/6 ÷ 3/7 x 5/9 =

    a. 6/5
    b. 1-1/6
    c. 135/129
    d. 175/162

99. For two points (4, 2) and (3, 5), what is the slope of a line going through both?

    a. −1
    b. 4
    c. −3
    d. 5

100. Which formula shown below is the correct formula for finding the area of the following polygon?

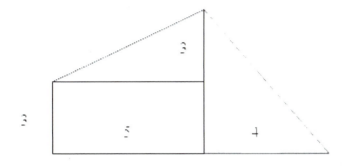

    a. (3 x 5)/2 + (3 x 5) + (4 x 6)/2
    b. 2(3 x 5) + (4 x 6)/2
    c. (3 x 5) + (3 x 6)/x + (4 x 6)
    d. (5 x 6) + (4 x 6)/2

Science Review

101. What is the name for any substance that stimulates the production of antibodies?
    a. collagen
    b. hemoglobin
    c. lymph
    d. antigen

102. Which of the following correctly lists the cellular hierarchy from the simplest to the most complex structure?
    a. tissue, cell, organ, organ system, organism
    b. organism, organ system, organ, tissue, cell
    c. organ system, organism, organ, tissue, cell
    d. cell, tissue, organ, organ system, organism

103. If a cell is placed in a hypertonic solution, what will happen to the cell?
    a. It will swell.
    b. It will shrink.
    c. It will stay the same.
    d. It does not affect the cell.

104. Which group of major parts and organs make up the immune system?
    a. lymphatic system, spleen, tonsils, thymus, and bone marrow
    b. brain, spinal cord, and nerve cells
    c. heart, veins, arteries, and capillaries
    d. nose, trachea, bronchial tubes, lungs, alveolus, and diaphragm

105. The rate of a chemical reaction depends on all of the following except
    a. temperature.
    b. surface area.
    c. presence of catalysts.
    d. amount of mass lost.

106. Which of the answer choices provided best defines the following statement?
        For a given mass and constant temperature, an inverse relationship exists between the volume and pressure of a gas?
    a. Ideal Gas Law
    b. Boyle's Law
    c. Charles' Law
    d. Stefan-Boltzmann Law

107. Which of the following statements correctly compares prokaryotic and eukaryotic cells?
    a. Prokaryotic cells have a true nucleus, eukaryotic cells do not.
    b. Both prokaryotic and eukaryotic cells have a membrane.
    c. Prokaryotic cells do not contain membrane-bound organelles, eukaryotic cells do.
    d. Prokaryotic cells are more complex than eukaryotic cells.

108. What is the role of ribosomes?
    a. make proteins
    b. waste removal
    c. transport
    d. storage

109. If an organism is *AaBb*, which of the following combinations in the gametes is impossible?
    a. AB
    b. aa
    c. aB
    d. Ab

110. What is the oxidation number of hydrogen in CaH_2?
    a. +1
    b. −1
    c. 0
    d. +2

111. Which hormone stimulates milk production in the breasts during lactation?
    a. norepinephrine
    b. antidiuretic hormone
    c. prolactin
    d. oxytocin

112. What is the typical result of mitosis in humans?
    a. two diploid cells
    b. two haploid cells
    c. four diploid cells
    d. four haploid cells

113. Which of the following does *not* exist as a diatomic molecule?
    a. boron
    b. fluorine
    c. oxygen
    d. nitrogen

114. Which of the following structures has the lowest blood pressure?
    a. arteries
    b. arteriole
    c. venule
    d. vein

115. How does water affect the temperature of a living thing?
    a. Water increases temperature.
    b. Water keeps temperature stable.
    c. Water decreases temperature.
    d. Water does not affect temperature.

116. What is another name for aqueous HI?
    a. hydroiodate acid
    b. hydrogen monoiodide
    c. hydrogen iodide
    d. hydriodic acid

117. Which of the heart chambers is the most muscular?
    a. left atrium
    b. right atrium
    c. left ventricle
    d. right ventricle

118. Which of the following is *not* a product of the Krebs cycle?
    a. carbon dioxide
    b. oxygen
    c. adenosine triphosphate (ATP)
    d. energy carriers

119. What is the name for the reactant that is entirely consumed by the reaction?
    a. limiting reactant
    b. reducing agent
    c. reaction intermediate
    d. reagent

120. Which part of the brain interprets sensory information?
    a. cerebrum
    b. hindbrain
    c. cerebellum
    d. medulla oblongata

121. What kind of bond connects sugar and phosphate in DNA?
    a. hydrogen
    b. ionic
    c. covalent
    d. overt

122. What is the mass (in grams) of 7.35 mol water?
    a. 10.7 g
    b. 18 g
    c. 132 g
    d. 180.6 g

123. Which of the following proteins is produced by cartilage?
    a. actin
    b. estrogen
    c. collagen
    d. myosin

124. How are lipids different than other organic molecules?
    a. They are indivisible.
    b. They are not water soluble.
    c. They contain zinc.
    d. They form long proteins.

125. Which of the following orbitals is the last to fill?
    a. 1s
    b . 3s
    c . 4p
    d. 6s

126. Which component of the nervous system is responsible for lowering the heart rate?
    a. central nervous system
    b. sympathetic nervous system
    c. parasympathetic nervous system
    d. distal nervous system

127. Which of the following is not a steroid?
    a. cholesterol
    b. estrogen
    c. testosterone
    d. hemoglobin

128. What is the name of the binary molecular compound NO5?
    a. nitro pentoxide
    b. ammonium pentoxide
    c. nitrogen pentoxide
    d. pentnitrogen oxide

129. In which of the following muscle types are the filaments arranged in a disorderly manner?
    a. cardiac
    b. smooth
    c. skeletal
    d. rough

130. Which hormone is produced by the pineal gland?
    a. insulin
    b. testosterone
    c. melatonin
    d. epinephrine

131. Which of the following is not true for all cells?
    a. Cells are the basic structures of any organism
    b. Cells can only reproduce from existing cells
    c. Cells are the smallest unit of any life form that carries the information needed for all life processes
    d. All cells are also called eukaryotes

132. What are the two types of cellular transport?
   a. Passive and diffusion
   b. Diffusion and active
   c. Active and passive
   d. Kinetic and active

133. Which of the following is not a state of matter?
   a. Gas
   b. Liquid
   c. Lattice
   d. Solid

134. What is the name for substances that cannot be broken down into simpler types of matter?
   a. Electron
   b. Molecules
   c. Nuclei
   d. Elements

135. Which of the following is the name for the study of the structure and shape of the human body?
   a. Physiology
   b. Anatomy
   c. Biology
   d. Genetics

136. Which of the following statements correctly describes a similarity or difference between rocks and minerals?
   a. Minerals may contain traces of organic compounds, while rocks do not.
   b. Rocks are classified by their formation and the minerals they contain, while minerals are classified by their chemical composition and physical properties.
   c. Both rocks and minerals can be polymorphs.
   d. Both rocks and minerals may contain mineraloids.

137. How many basic tissue types does a human have?
   a. 4
   b. 6
   c. 12
   d. 23

138. What does aerobic mean?
   a. In the presence of oxygen
   b. Calorie-burning
   c. Heated
   d. Anabolic

139. Which of the following is NOT one of the five major physical properties of minerals?
   a. Chemical composition
   b. Hardness
   c. Luster
   d. Streak

140. Which of the following factors directly contributes to soil erosion?
   a. Air pollution from cars and factories
   b. Use of pesticides
   c. Deforestation and overgrazing
   d. Water pollution caused by excess sedimentation

141. Which of the following is the name for the study of how parts of the body function?
   a. Physiology
   b. Anatomy
   c. Biology
   d. Genetics

142. Which of these minerals would have the lowest score on the Mohs scale?
   a. Gypsum
   b. Fluorite
   c. Talc
   d. Diamond

143. Which of the following organ systems has the purpose of producing movement through contraction?
   a. Skeletal
   b. Muscular
   c. Cardiovascular
   d. Respiratory

144. Which of the following lists places several phases of the sedimentary cycle in the correct order?
   a. Erosion, weathering, transportation, deposition
   b. Weathering, erosion, deposition, transportation
   c. Weathering, deposition, erosion, transportation
   d. Weathering, erosion, transportation, deposition

145. Water is likely to have the shortest residence time in which of the following types of reservoirs?
   a. A glacier
   b. A lake
   c. A river
   d. The atmosphere

146. When an earthquake occurs, the "shaking" that is observed results directly from:
    a. Static deformation.
    b. Seismic waves.
    c. Compression waves.
    d. Continental drift.

147. An atom with an electrical charge is called a(n):
    a. Electron
    b. Ion
    c. Molecule
    d. Enzyme

148. When water changes directly from a solid to a gas, skipping the liquid state, this is called:
    a. Evapotranspiration.
    b. Condensation.
    c. Sublimation.
    d. Runoff.

149. What are the two types of measurement important in science?
    a. quantitative and numerical
    b. qualitative and descriptive
    c. numerical and scientific
    d. quantitative and qualitative

150. Which of the following is a true statement about the Earth's oceans?
    a. Oceans comprise about 50 percent of the Earth's surface.
    b. The deepest point in the ocean is about 6,000 meters below sea level.
    c. The ocean is divided geographically into four areas: the Atlantic, Pacific, Mediterranean, and Indian.
    d. The ocean's salinity is usually between 34 and 35 parts per thousand, or 200 parts per million.

151. Approximately 96.5 percent of seawater is comprised of:
    a. Hydrogen and sodium.
    b. Hydrogen and oxygen.
    c. Oxygen and sodium.
    d. Chlorine and sodium

152. Which of the below is the best definition for the term circulation?
    a. The transport of oxygen and other nutrients to the tissues via the cardiovascular system
    b. The force exerted by blood against a unit area of the blood vessel walls
    c. The branching air passageways inside the lungs
    d. The process of breathing in

153. Which of the following techniques is NOT a radiometric dating process?
   a. Potassium-argon dating
   b. Stratigraphic dating
   c. Uranium-lead dating
   d. Chlorine-36 dating

154. What is the typical way a solid would turn to a liquid and then to a gas?
   a. Vaporization then melting
   b. Melting then freezing
   c. Vaporization then freezing
   d. Melting then vaporization

155. Which of the following is an example of an absolute age?
   a. A fossil is 37 million years old.
   b. A rock is less than 100,000 years old.
   c. An organic artifact is between 5,000 and 10,000 years old.
   d. All of the above

156. Which of the following is true?
   a. Mass and weight are the same thing
   b. Mass is the quantity of matter an object has
   c. Mass equals twice the weight of an object
   d. Mass equals half the weight of an object

157. Which of the following life forms appeared first on Earth?
   a. Eukaryotes
   b. Arthropods
   c. Prokaryotes
   d. Amphibians

158. Which law of classical thermodynamics states that energy can neither be created nor destroyed?
   a. Zeroth
   b. First
   c. Second
   d. Third

159. Which organ system includes the spleen?
   a. Endocrine
   b. Lymphatic
   c. Respiratory
   d. Digestive

160. The formula for calculating kinetic energy is:
   a. ½ mv2.
   b. ½ mv.
   c. mgh.
   d. mgv.

Answer Key and Explanations

Verbal Review

1. A: The best synonym for *ominous* as it is used in this sentence is "threatening." An ominous symptom, for instance, is one that suggests the presence of serious disease. The word *emboldening* means "making bold." A patient who is regaining strength might be emboldened to try new and more difficult activities. The word *destructive* means "causing damage, chaos, or loss." A destructive condition or behavior has a negative effect on the patient's health. The word *insightful* means "thoughtful or provocative." As a health practitioner, you should try to be insightful so that you can come up with creative solutions to your patients' problems.

2. A: The closest meaning for the word *occluded* as it is used in this sentence is "closed." Occluded means "blocked or obstructed." The word is commonly used to describe arteries that no longer allow the passage of blood. The word *deformed* means "misshapen or out of the normal shape." Any deformed body part is a cause for concern. The word *engorged* means "overfull, especially of blood or food." The organs of the body may become engorged when they are infected or diseased. *Enlarged* means "made larger."

3. D: The word *precipitous* as it is used this sentence means "steep." Doctors will often refer to a precipitous change in blood pressure. In general, precipitous changes are dangerous to the health. The word *detached* means "unconnected or aloof." A common example is a detached retina, a condition in which part of the eye becomes disconnected, and vision is damaged. The word *sordid* means "dirty" or "vile." The word *encompassed* means "surrounded or entirely contained within." For instance, a doctor might describe a treatment protocol as encompassing all aspects of the patient's life.

4. C: The word *vital* as it is used this sentence means "essential." Medical workers will often refer to a patient's vital signs, meaning blood pressure, heart rate, and temperature. The word *recommended* means "preferred by some authority." The recommended course of treatment is the one outlined and prescribed by a doctor. The word *discouraged* means "disappointed and doubtful of success." Health-care workers should try to prevent patients from becoming discouraged, since this can further diminish quality of life and chances of recovery. The word *sufficient* means "having enough to accomplish the necessary task." As an example, a doctor might inquire to make sure that a patient is receiving sufficient fluids or food.

5. C: The word *distended* as it is used in this sentence means "swollen." Doctors will often refer to a distended abdomen, which accompanies gassiness or bloating. The word *concave* means "shaped like the inside of a bowl." Many structures of the human body, for instance the inside of the ear and the arch of the foot, are described as concave. A distended body part may be *sore*, but it is not necessarily so. A distended artery, for instance, may have no accompanying pain. Also, though a distended body part may be *empty*, this is not always the

- 28 -

case. In cases of starvation, the stomach may become distended; however, other body parts may become distended from being full to excess.

6. B: The word *overt* as it is used in this sentence means "apparent." Overt signs are those that can be seen by someone other than the person who is experiencing them. A rash is an overt sign; a stomachache is not. The word *concealed* means "hidden." Concealed signs cannot be perceived with the senses; a rise in blood pressure, for instance, is a concealed sign of illness. The word *expert*, used as an adjective, means "knowledgeable about a particular subject." When dealing with an unfamiliar situation, for instance, a doctor might call in an expert practitioner. The word *delectable* means "tasty or delicious."

7. A: The word *recur* as it is used in this sentence means "occur again." Doctors often refer to the recurrence of a disease or symptom. In some cases, the recurrence of a disease indicates that the treatment used in the past was ineffective. *Recur* has the same root as *occur*, with the prefix *re-*, meaning "back or again." To *survive* means "to remain alive." To *collect* means "to bring together into one place." To *desist* means "to cease or stop doing something." A doctor might advise a patient to desist from a certain behavior in order to improve his or her health.

8. D: The word *endogenous* as it is used in this sentence means "growing from within." Doctors occasionally refer to endogenous cholesterol, which comes from inside the body rather than from the diet. *Contagious* means "capable of spreading from person to person." A person with a contagious disease needs to be kept away from other people. Often, diseases are only contagious for a limited time. *Continuous* means "proceeding on without stopping." If a patient is suffering from continuous back pain, for instance, he or she is experiencing the pain at all times.

9. B: The word *lethargic* as it is used in this sentence means "sluggish." Lethargy is a symptom of many forms of illness. It is also a side effect of chemotherapy. *Nauseous* means "sickened, or suffering from an upset stomach." Nausea is a common side effect of chemotherapy as well; it is just not the one described in this sentence. *Contagious* means "capable of spreading from person to person." Many viral and bacterial infections are contagious. *Elated* means "ecstatic," or "wildly happy." It is usually a good thing when a patient is elated, although manic-depressive patients may alternate between excessive elation and near-suicidal sadness.

10. B: The word *site* as it is used in this sentence means "location." Doctors will often refer to the site of an injection or a planned surgery. A *syringe* is "the device used to inject or withdraw fluid from the body." Medical personnel who specialize in withdrawing blood from patients are called phlebotomists. An *artery* is "a blood vessel that carries blood away from the heart to nourish the rest of the body." Although the site to which the author is referring in this sentence is a *hole*, it will not always be so. For this reason, "hole" cannot be the best definition for *site*.

11. A: The word *exposure* as it is used in this sentence means "laying open." The most common usage of this term is in reference to the sun, although exposure to toxic chemicals is also a major health concern. A doctor will often ask a patient to limit his or her exposure to some environmental element. *Prohibition* is "the act of forbidding." Often, a doctor will

place a prohibition on certain behaviors or foods if they are believed to adversely affect health. The words *connection* and *dislike* have no relation to exposure.

12. D: The word *holistic* as it is used in this sentence means "concerned with the whole rather than the parts." Doctors try to consider the patient's health from a holistic perspective; that is, they try to improve health in its entirety rather than to eliminate specific symptoms. The word *insensitive* means "not responsive." The word *ignorant* means "lacking knowledge." Health-care workers cannot be ignorant of the latest findings and information in their field. The word *specialized* means "adapted to or trained in a specific discipline or task." Because of the technological complexity of modern medical practice, most careers in health care are specialized.

13. C: The word *symmetric* as it is used in this sentence means "occurring in corresponding parts at the same time." Some illnesses will cause symmetric rashes, meaning that both the right and left sides of the body are afflicted with similarly shaped inflammation. The word *scabbed* means "covered with wounds." The word *geometric* is used to describe "things that resemble the classic geometric shapes, such as the circle, square, or triangle." On occasion, a doctor may use this word to describe the pattern of a wound or rash.

14. C: The word *volume* as it is used in this sentence means "quantity." Doctors will refer to an increase in the volume of urine or some other body product as an indication of health. Volume is calculated as length × width × height (or depth); it is a three-dimensional measure. *Length*, on the other hand, is "a two-dimensional measure of distance." *Quality* means "degree of excellence." Quantity can be measured in any kind of units. *Loudness* might be the right answer if *volume* were being used in a different way, as "the relative power of a sound." In this sentence, however, the word is not being used to describe a sound.

15. C: The word "precipitous" means "steep."

16. B: The word "obscure" means "unclear" and "difficult to understand."

17. C: The word "remiss" means "negligent or forgetful."

18. B: Brandish means to wave menacingly.

19. A: Besotted means infatuated

20. A: Vicinity means neighborhood.

21. B: Famished means hungry.

22. A: Enamored means fascinated.

23. D: Dissect means to analyze as used in the provided sentence.

24. A: Apprized means appreciated.

25. B: *Pale* is an exact synonym for *pallid*, which in this context means that he lacks a healthy skin color. This could indicate infection or disease. Two of these answers are related terms but not synonyms. *Sallow* is similar, as it means, "lacking the warm skin color indicating good health." *Sickly* denotes "chronically or regularly suffering from poor health," which is not necessarily true if a person has pallid skin. *Sanguine* is an antonym for pallid and pale; the word has several meanings, but as related to skin color it means, "possessing a healthy reddish skin color."

26. C: *Diurnal* is a synonym for daily, which means "done, taking place, appearing, or produced every day." *Continuous* implies nonstop administration without interruptions. *Nightly* is a near antonym for diurnal and daily; it means "occurring during the night." *Parenteral* administration occurs through injection, a drip feed, or implantation.

27. D: *Bewilderment* is one synonym for confusion, which has several meanings of application here. *Confusion* could mean that the patient is in either a state of mental uncertainty or an emotional state of embarrassment. *Agitation* is a related word, but it means that the person is in a state of either (1) wild emotion or activity, or (2) uneasiness in anticipation of trouble. *Certitude* is a near antonym, because it means that the person is in a state of mind in which they are free from doubt. *Indifference* denotes a lack of interest or desire, which could accompany confusion.

28. A: As a verb, *clot* is a synonym for coagulate, which means, "to cause a liquid to thicken into a semisolid mass or substance resembling jelly." *Deliquesce* is a near antonym meaning, "to go from a solid to a liquid state." *Solidify* is a related but less specific term meaning that something (1) becomes firm or solid, or (2) takes on a definite form. Ideas about how to treat a patient can eventually solidify, for example. As a verb form, *separate* has several definitions, the closest one applicable in this instance being "to set or force apart." After collection, blood separates into the coagulated clot and the clear serum.

29. B: *Cadenced* is another word for *rhythmic*, which means that something "has or occurs with a perceptible regularity in rise and fall of sound." Cadenced breathing would be considered "normal," but the latter is a more general word for terms like "typical, average, ordinary, or sane." *Regular* is a related word with several meanings, the closest being that something follows a set pattern. *Irregular* would be an antonym to regular.

30. C: *Impending* is a synonym for *imminent*, which suggests signs of immediate occurrence or that a condition will appear or take place soon. Urgency is implied. *Portentous* is a related term meaning that something "is or shows signs of upcoming evil or calamity." *Eventual* simply implies that something will occur at a later time, and *prophetic* means "predictive or being a sign of a later course of action."

31. C: *Obscure* and *ambiguous* can both mean, "having a deliberately veiled or uncertain meaning." Two of the other choices are related words, but they do not imply intent. *Confounding* means, "thrown into a state of mental uncertainty." *Unclear* means, "not clearly expressed, seen, or understood." *Straightforward* is a near antonym of *obscure* and indicates that something has been done or said in a direct and honest manner.

32. D: Both *compliance* and *deference* describe a state of willingness or readiness to yield to others' desires. *Complaisance* and *acquiescence* are related terms. *Complaisance* is very

similar in that it means, "a desire to please and carry out the wishes of others." *Acquiescence* means "agreement in a passive manner." *Defiance* is an antonym meaning "open or hostile disobedience."

33. B: *Fraught* is the only true synonym for *rife*, which means that something is found widely or frequently. *Overloaded* is related but implies an excess load or burden. *Devoid* is an antonym meaning, "utterly lacking in something." In this sentence, *transcribed* acts as a verb, not as an adverb like the other words, and means to "copy, expand from notes, or translate something." Healthcare professionals regularly transcribe gathered information onto the patient's chart, but the word is unrelated to "rife."

34. D: *Dilemma* is the only synonym for *quandary*, which means, "a situation in which a person has to decide between two or more unsatisfactory choices." For example, the doctor might have given her treatment choices such as lumpectomy versus mastectomy. *Impasse* is a related term meaning, "a point at which progress cannot occur or agreement reached." Anna does need to make a decision, which is a "stance determined after consideration," but the word is distinct from *quandary*. *Heartbreak* is also an unrelated term, meaning "intense grief."

35. C: *Disavowed* and *disclaimed* are synonyms, both meaning "denied responsibility for, knowledge of, or association with." *Rejected* is related, but means, "denied, declined, or discarded." *Acknowledged* is an antonym indicating formal recognition of something. Approved is somewhat related to *acknowledged*, not *disavowed*; if used in this sentence, it would mean, "gave official recognition as acceptable."

36. C: The sentence reads, "Your brain <u>filters</u> [your nose] out," which means your brain ignores it.

37. B: Only choice B reflects the meaning of the term "retina," which is a part of the eye's anatomy.

38. B: The final sentence reads, "Your brain works hard to make the world look continuous." It follows that visual perception is an active process, not a passive one, making choice B the best answer.

39. A: If the reader follows the instructions given in the paragraph, the O and X in the middle of the passage can be used to demonstrate the blind spot in the visual field. Choice A is the best answer.

40. B: The passage explains the way that visual perception works. Choice B is the best answer.

41. D: Much of the information in the passage is provided to show examples of how the brain fills in gaps in the visual field. Choice D is the best answer.

42. A: The author of the passage mentions the nose to demonstrate how the brain filters information out of the visual field. Choice A is the best answer.

43. B: Choice B can be inferred from the second paragraph. The paragraph states that the brain filters out information, which means that the brain does not perceive all activity in the visual field.

44. B: Choice B, "ODD is a complex condition" is the best answer out of the four given. It is the only choice that can be inferred from the passage as a whole.

45. A: Choice A is the best choice. Oppositional means uncooperative.

46. B: Choice B is the best interpretation of paragraph one. The passage states that many people exhibit ODD symptoms from time to time.

47. C: Feed into in this sentence means to encourage oppositional behavior.

48. C: Someone with low frustration tolerance has a difficult time tolerating or dealing with frustration.

49. C: This passage is meant to inform the reader about ODD. Choice C is the best choice.

50. C: While some of these answer choices may contribute to ODD, the passage mentions only choice C severe or unpredictable punishment.

51. A: The only statement directly supported by the passage is choice A.

52. B: As used in this passage, the word "parasite" means an organism that lives on or in another organism, Choice B. Choice A and C are obviously wrong, since the passage mentions nothing of Paris or insects. Choice D is another definition for "parasite," but does not fit the context of the word used in this passage.

53. C: According to the description of Roundworms, they can live in the subcutaneous tissue of humans, Choice C. Choices A, B, and D describe where protozoa live and how they are transmitted.

54. D: According to the first paragraph, protozoa are transmitted through food and water contaminated by fecal matter. It can then be inferred that clean sanitary conditions will prevent the spread of protozoa, Choice D. Choice A is an incorrect inference because the passage discusses both larval and adult forms of parasites that infect humans. Choice B is an incorrect inference, since the first paragraph states that protozoa are transmitted by mosquitoes. Choice C is an incorrect inference because the second paragraph is about worms that infect humans.

55. D: To answer this question, you will need to verify all three statements in the passage. All three of these statements are true and are supported by the passage.

56. D: Since the passage describes superstitions from days gone by about treating asthma, answer choice D is the correct one. Answer choice A, asthma in the United States, is incorrect because even though that is mentioned in the first sentence, it is not the main idea. Answer choice B, methods of treating asthma, is not the best choice since it is vague about whether the methods are current or from long ago. Answer choice C, old wives tales, might have been a choice if old wives' tales had been mentioned in the passage, but it is not the best choice.

57. A: The reader can infer from the opening sentence that if so many people have asthma today, many would probably have had asthma long ago as well. Even though the environment today is different than it was long ago, people would still have suffered from the condition. The sentence explains why people long ago may have needed to try homemade methods of treating the condition.

58. B: The purpose of the passage is to describe different measures that people took for asthma long ago, before the advent of modern medicine. Answer choice A, herbal remedies, is incorrect because the majority of the "medicine" described in the passage is not herbal. The passage does not, as in answer choice C, define superstitions. Nor does it praise modern medicine, as answer choice D suggests.

59. A: Of all the choices listed, only answer choice A is an example of misusing a drug. It is listed as one of the ways that drugs are misused in the middle of the passage. Taking more or less of a prescription drug than the amount that the doctor ordered can be harmful to one's health. The other answer choices are not examples of misuse, nor do they appear in the passage. Make sure all of your answer choices are based on the passage given rather than information you may know or assume from other sources.

60. D: The passage does not say that ALL drugs add longevity. It says that drugs that are healthy and used properly add longevity. The word *all* makes the statement untrue.

Mathematics Review

61. D: This is a simple addition problem. Start with the ones column (on the right). Add the figures 6+1, 3+0, 2+3 to get the answer 537.

62. C: This is a simple addition problem with carrying. Start with the ones column and add 7+4, write down the 1 and add the 1 to the digits in the tens column. Now add 0+6+1. Write down the 7. Now add 3+8 and write down the 1. Add the 1 to the thousands column. Add 4+1+1 and write the 6 to get the answer 6171.

63. B: Simply substitute the given values for *a* and *b* and perform the required operations.

64. A: This is a subtraction problem which involves borrowing. Start with the ones column. Since 7 can't be subtracted from 6, borrow ten from the tens column. Cross out the 5 and make it a 4. Now subtract 7 from 16. Write down 9. Move to the tens column Since 6 can't be subtracted from 4, borrow ten from the hundreds column. Cross out the 3 and make it a 2. 14-6 = 8. Now subtract 1 from 2 and write down 1 to get 189.

65. B: This is a subtraction problem which also involves borrowing. Start with the ones column. Since 7 can't be subtracted from 6, borrow ten from the tens column. Cross out the 0 and make it a 9. Cross out the 2 in the hundreds column and make it a 2. Now subtract 7 from 16. Write down 9. Move to the tens column. Subtract 8 from 9 and write down 1. Move to the hundreds column. Since you can't subtract 4 from 3, borrow ten from the thousands column. Cross out the 5 and make it a 4. 12-4= 8. Now subtract 3 from 4 and write down 1 to get 1819.

66. C: This problem is solved by finding *x* in this equation: $34/80 = x/100$.

67. A: This is a multiplication problem with 0. Start with the 7 in 17 and multiply it by each of the digits at the top 7 x 7. Write down the 9 and place the 4 in the tens column. 7 x 0 is 0. Add the 4. 7 x 7 is 49. The top line will read 4949. Now multiply 1 by 7. Write down the 7. 1 x 0 is 0 and 1 x 7 is 7. The bottom line will read 707.Add these together with the 7 in the tens column and the answer will be 12,019.

68. A: This is a simple division problem. Divide the 7 into 9. It goes in 1 time. Write 1 above the 9 and subtract 7 from 9 to get 2. Bring down the 1 and place it beside the 2. Divide 7 into 21. It goes in 3 times. Divide 7 into 7. It goes 1 time. .

69. D: To solve this problem, work backwards. That is, perform FOIL on each answer choice until you derive the original expression.

70. A: To change this fraction into a decimal, divide 100 into 38. 100 goes into 38 .38 times.

71. C: This is a simple addition problem. Line up the decimals so that they are all in the same place in the equation, and see that there is a 6 by itself in the hundredths column. Then add the tenths column: 8+3to get 11. Write down the 1 and carry the 1. Add the ones column: 6+1 plus the carried 1. Write down 8. Then write down the 1.

72. A: A set of six numbers with an average of 4 must have a collective sum of 24. The two numbers that average 2 will add up to 4, so the remaining numbers must add up to 20. The average of these four numbers can be calculated: 20/4 = 5.

73. C: Count from the 3: tenths, hundredths, thousandths.

74. A: This is a simple subtraction problem with decimals. Line up the decimals and subtract 9 from 8. Since this can't be done, borrow 10 from the 5. Cross out the 5 and make it 4. Now subtract 9 from 18 to get 9. Subtract 3 from 4 and get 1. Place the decimal point before the 1.

75. D: Simple Multiplication.

76. A: To add fractions, ensure that the denominator (the number on the bottom) is the same. Since it is not, change them both to 56ths. 1/8 equals 7/56. 3/7 equals 24/56. Now add the whole numbers: 3+6 = 9 and the fractions 31/56.

77. C: To subtract fractions, ensure that the denominator (the number on the bottom) is the same. Since it is not, change them both to 14ths. 1/7 = 2/14; 1/2 = 7/14. The equation now looks like this: $4\frac{2}{14} - 2\frac{7}{14}$. Change the 4 to 3 and add 14 to the numerator (the top number) so that the fractions can be subtracted. The equation now looks like this: $3\frac{16}{14}$ $2\frac{7}{14}$.

Subtract: $1\frac{9}{14}$

78. A: To multiply mixed numbers, first create improper fractions. Multiply the whole number by the denominator, then add the numerator. $1\frac{1}{4}$ becomes $\frac{5}{4}$; $3\frac{2}{5}$ becomes $\frac{17}{5}$; $1\frac{2}{3}$ becomes $\frac{5}{3}$.

The problem will look like this: $\frac{5}{4} \times \frac{17}{5} \times \frac{5}{3} = \frac{425}{60} = 7\frac{5}{60} = 7\frac{1}{12}$.

79. C: There are 12 inches in a foot and 3 feet in a yard. Four and a half yards is equal to 162 inches. To determine the number of 3-inche segments, divide 162 by 3.

80. C: Divide the numerator and denominator by 14.

81. A: Write .36, and then move the decimal two places. Add the percent sign.

82. C: 10% of 900 is 90. Multiply 90 by 4 to find 40%.

83. A: If it takes 3 people 3 1/3 days to do the job, then it would take one person 10 days: 3 × 3 1/3 = 10. Thus, it would take 2 people 5 days, and one day of work for two people would complete 1/5 of the job.

84. A: Divide 40 by 8 to get 5. Multiply 5 by 3 to get 15.

85. B: Rewrite the problem as 25 X 0.06 and solve.

86. D: Divide 4 by 16 (not 16 by 4) and multiply by 100 to provide answer in % form as requested.

87. C: Since 4 is the same as 2^2, $4^6 = 2^{12}$. When dividing exponents with the same base, simply subtract the exponent in the denominator from the exponent in the numerator.

88. D: To solve, rewrite the percent as a fraction: 30/100 .
Then reduce the fraction.

89. C: To change a percent to a decimal, remove the percent sign and move the decimal two spaces to the left.

90. A: To solve, add 6 a and 2a, then subtract 4a.

91. B: Substitute the given values and solve. Resolve the parenthetical operations first.

92. D: To solve, combine like terms, ensuring that the subtraction sign is notice and positive/negative signs are changed accordingly:
$x^2 - x^2 = 0$; $-3x - 3x = 6x$; $-3 - 3 = -6$

93. B: To solve, get the variable (y) by itself:
$4x = 21 - 5$; $4y = 16$; $y = 4$

94. B: To solve, first do the multiplication on each side of the equation: $3x + 42 = 4x = 36$. Then get like terms on opposite sides of the equation: $x = 6$

95. A: Convert 20% to the fraction 1/5, then multiply by 12/5. The resulting fraction, 12/25, must have both numerator and denominator multiplied by 4 to become a percentage.

96. D: The perimeter is found by adding all sides of a figure. In the case of a rectangle, two of the sides are going to be equal in length, so if the width is 10 feet and the height 15 feet, formula would be 10 + 10 + 15 + 15, or 2(10) + 2(15).

97. B: The students making A's and B's represent 70% of the student body. If 53 students make D's, that is approximately 10% of the student body, leaving the remaining 20% to make C's.

98. D: The test-taker must follow the order of operations, which in this case is simply left to right with multiplication and division. (5/6)*(7/3) = (35/18). (35/18)*(5/9) = 175/162.

99. C: The equation for finding the slope is $(y2 - y1)/(x2 - x1)$. With the points provided, the equation becomes (5-2)/(3-4), or (3)/(-1): -3.

100. A: To find the area of the parallelogram, the area of each shape must be determined and then added together. The area of the smaller triangle is (3 x 5)/2. The area of the

rectangle is (3 x 5), and the area of the larger triangle is (4 x 6)/2. This leaves only the formula provided in answer choice A.

Science Review

101. D: The name for a substance that stimulates the production of antibodies is an *antigen*. An antigen is any substance perceived by the immune system as dangerous. When the body senses an antigen, it produces an antibody. *Collagen* is one of the components of bone, tendon, and cartilage. It is a spongy protein that can be turned into gelatin by boiling. *Hemoglobin* is the part of red blood cells that carries oxygen. In order for the blood to carry enough oxygen to the cells of the body, there has to be a sufficient amount of hemoglobin. *Lymph* is a near-transparent fluid that performs a number of functions in the body: It removes bacteria from tissues, replaces lymphocytes in the blood, and moves fat away from the small intestine. Lymph contains white blood cells. As you can see, some of the questions in the vocabulary section will require technical knowledge.

102. D: The cellular hierarchy starts with the cell, the simplest structure, and progresses to organisms, the most complex structures.

103. B: A hypertonic solution is a solution with a higher particle concentration than in the cell, and consequently lower water content than in the cell. Water moves from the cell to the solution, causing the cell to experience water loss and shrink.

104. A: The immune system consists of the lymphatic system, spleen, tonsils, thymus and bone marrow.

105. D: The rate at which a chemical reaction occurs does not depend on the amount of mass lost, since the law of conservation of mass (or matter) states that in a chemical reaction there is no loss of mass.

106. B: Boyle's law states that for a constant mass and temperature, pressure and volume are related inversely to one another: $PV = c$, where c = constant.

107. C: Prokaryotic cells are simpler cells that do not have membrane-bound organelles, whereas eukaryotic cells have several membrane-bound organelles.

108. A: A ribosome is a structure of eukaryotic cells that makes proteins

109. B: It is impossible for an *AaBb* organism to have the *aa* combination in the gametes. It is impossible for each letter to be used more than one time, so it would be impossible for the lowercase *a* to appear twice in the gametes. It would be possible, however, for *Aa* to appear in the gametes, since there is one uppercase *A* and one lowercase *a*. Gametes are the cells involved in sexual reproduction. They are germ cells.

110. B: The oxidation number of the hydrogen in CaH_2 is −1. The oxidation number is the positive or negative charge of a monoatomic ion. In other words, the oxidation number is the numerical charge on an ion. An ion is a charged version of an element. Oxidation number is often referred to as oxidation state. Oxidation number is sometimes used to describe the number of electrons that must be added or removed from an atom in order to convert the atom to its elemental form.

111. C: *Prolactin* stimulates the production of breast milk during lactation. *Norepinephrine* is a hormone and neurotransmitter secreted by the adrenal gland that regulates heart rate, blood pressure, and blood sugar. *Antidiuretic hormone* is produced by the hypothalamus and secreted by the pituitary gland. It regulates the concentration of urine and triggers the contractions of the arteries and capillaries. *Oxytocin* is a hormone secreted by the pituitary gland that makes it easier to eject milk from the breast and manages the contractions of the uterus during labor.

112. A: The typical result of mitosis in humans is two diploid cells. *Mitosis* is the division of a body cell into two daughter cells. Each of the two produced cells has the same set of chromosomes as the parent. A diploid cell contains both sets of homologous chromosomes. A haploid cell contains only one set of chromosomes, which means that it only has a single set of genes.

113. A: Boron does not exist as a diatomic molecule. The other possible answer choices, fluorine, oxygen, and nitrogen, all exist as diatomic molecules. A diatomic molecule always appears in nature as a pair: The word *diatomic* means "having two atoms." With the exception of astatine, all of the halogens are diatomic. Chemistry students often use the mnemonic BrINClHOF (pronounced "brinkelhoff") to remember all of the diatomic elements: bromine, iodine, nitrogen, chlorine, hydrogen, oxygen, and fluorine. Note that not all of these diatomic elements are halogens.

114. D: Of the given structures, veins have the lowest blood pressure. *Veins* carry oxygen-poor blood from the outlying parts of the body to the heart. An *artery* carries oxygen-rich blood from the heart to the peripheral parts of the body. An *arteriole* extends from an artery to a capillary. A *venule* is a tiny vein that extends from a capillary to a larger vein.

115. B: Water stabilizes the temperature of living things. The ability of warm-blooded animals, including human beings, to maintain a constant internal temperature is known as *homeostasis*. Homeostasis depends on the presence of water in the body. Water tends to minimize changes in temperature because it takes a while to heat up or cool down. When the human body gets warm, the blood vessels dilate and blood moves away from the torso and toward the extremities. When the body gets cold, blood concentrates in the torso. This is the reason why hands and feet tend to get especially cold in cold weather.

116. D: Hydriodic acid is another name for aqueous HI. In an aqueous solution, the solvent is water. Hydriodic acid is a polyatomic ion, meaning that it is composed of two or more elements. When this solution has an increased amount of oxygen, the -*ate* suffix on the first word is converted to -*ic*. This process can be quite complex, so you should carefully review this material before your exam.

117. C: Of the four heart chambers, the left ventricle is the most muscular. When it contracts, it pushes blood out to the organs and extremities of the body. The right ventricle pushes blood into the lungs. The atria, on the other hand, receive blood from the outlying parts of the body and transport it into the ventricles. The basic process works as follows: Oxygen-poor blood fills the right atrium and is pumped into the right ventricle, from which it is pumped into the pulmonary artery and on to the lungs. In the lungs, this blood is oxygenated. The blood then reenters the heart at the left atrium, which when full pumps

into the left ventricle. When the left ventricle is full, blood is pushed into the aorta and on to the organs and extremities of the body.

118. B: Oxygen is not one of the products of the Krebs cycle. The *Krebs cycle* is the second stage of cellular respiration. In this stage, a sequence of reactions converts pyruvic acid into carbon dioxide. This stage of cellular respiration produces the phosphate compounds that provide most of the energy for the cell. The Krebs cycle is also known as the citric acid cycle or the tricarboxylic acid cycle.

119. A: A limiting reactant is entirely used up by the chemical reaction. Limiting reactants control the extent of the reaction and determine the quantity of the product. A reducing agent is a substance that reduces the amount of another substance by losing electrons. A reagent is any substance used in a chemical reaction. Some of the most common reagents in the laboratory are sodium hydroxide and hydrochloric acid. The behavior and properties of these substances are known, so they can be effectively used to produce predictable reactions in an experiment.

120. A: The *cerebrum* is the part of the brain that interprets sensory information. It is the largest part of the brain. The cerebrum is divided into two hemispheres, connected by a thin band of tissue called the corpus callosum. The *cerebellum* is positioned at the back of the head, between the brain stem and the cerebrum. It controls both voluntary and involuntary movements. The *medulla oblongata* forms the base of the brain. This part of the brain is responsible for blood flow and breathing, among other things.

121. C: The sugar and phosphate in DNA are connected by covalent bonds. A *covalent bond* is formed when atoms share electrons. It is very common for atoms to share pairs of electrons. An *ionic bond* is created when one or more electrons are transferred between atoms. *Ionic bonds*, also known as *electrovalent bonds*, are formed between ions with opposite charges. There is no such thing as an *overt bond* in chemistry.

122. C: The mass of 7.35 mol water is 132 grams. You should be able to find the mass of various chemical compounds when you are given the number of mols. The information required to perform this function is included on the periodic table. To solve this problem, find the molecular mass of water by finding the respective weights of hydrogen and oxygen. Remember that water contains two hydrogen molecules and one oxygen molecule. The molecular mass of hydrogen is roughly 1, and the molecular mass of oxygen is roughly 16. A molecule of water, then, has approximately 18 grams of mass. Multiply this by 7.35 mol, and you will obtain the answer 132.3, which is closest to answer choice C.

123. C: *Collagen* is the protein produced by cartilage. Bone, tendon, and cartilage are all mainly composed of collagen. *Actin* and *myosin* are the proteins responsible for muscle contractions. Actin makes up the thinner fibers in muscle tissue, while myosin makes up the thicker fibers. Myosin is the most numerous cell protein in human muscle. *Estrogen* is one of the steroid hormones produced mainly by the ovaries. Estrogen motivates the menstrual cycle and the development of female sex characteristics.

124. B: Unlike other organic molecules, lipids are not water soluble. Lipids are typically composed of carbon and hydrogen. Three common types of lipid are fats, waxes, and oils. Indeed, lipids usually feel oily when you touch them. All living cells are primarily composed of lipids, carbohydrates, and proteins. Some examples of fats are lard, corn oil, and butter.

Some examples of waxes are beeswax and carnauba wax. Some examples of steroids are cholesterol and ergosterol.

125. D: Of these orbitals, the last to fill is 6s. Orbitals fill in the following order: 1s, 2s, 2p, 3s, 3p, 4s, 3d, 4p, 5s, 4d, 5p, 6s, 4f, 5d, 6p, 7s, 5f, 6d, and 7p. The number is the orbital number, and the letter is the sublevel identification. Sublevel s has one orbital and can hold a maximum of two electrons. Sublevel p has three orbitals and can hold a maximum of six electrons. Sublevel d has five orbitals and can hold a maximum of 10 electrons. Sublevel f has seven orbitals and can hold a maximum of 14 electrons.

126. C: The parasympathetic nervous system is responsible for lowering the heart rate. It slows down the heart rate, dilates the blood vessels, and increases the secretions of the digestive system. The central nervous system is composed of the brain and the spinal cord. The sympathetic nervous system is a part of the autonomic nervous system; its role is to oppose the actions taken by the parasympathetic nervous system. So, the sympathetic nervous system accelerates the heart, contracts the blood vessels, and decreases the secretions of the digestive system.

127. D: *Hemoglobin* is not a steroid. It is a protein that helps to move oxygen from the lungs to the various body tissues. Steroids can be either synthetic chemicals used to reduce swelling and inflammation or sex hormones produced by the body. *Cholesterol* is the most abundant steroid in the human body. It is necessary for the creation of bile, though it can be dangerous if the levels in the body become too high. *Estrogen* is a female steroid produced by the ovaries (in females), testes (in males), placenta, and adrenal cortex. It contributes to adolescent sexual development, menstruation, mood, lactation, and aging. *Testosterone* is the main hormone produced by the testes; it is responsible for the development of adult male sex characteristics.

128. C: Nitrogen pentoxide is the name of the binary molecular compound NO_5. The format given in answer choice C is appropriate when dealing with two nonmetals. A prefix is used to denote the number of atoms of each element. Note that when there are seven atoms of a given element, the prefix *hepta-* is used instead of the usual *septa-*. Also, when the first atom in this kind of binary molecular compound is single, it does not need to be given the prefix *mono-*.

129. B: Smooth muscle tissue is said to be arranged in a disorderly fashion because it is not striated like the other two types of muscle: cardiac and skeletal. Striations are lines that can only be seen with a microscope. *Smooth* muscle is typically found in the supporting tissues of hollow organs and blood vessels. *Cardiac* muscle is found exclusively in the heart; it is responsible for the contractions that pump blood throughout the body. *Skeletal* muscle, by far the most preponderant in the body, controls the movements of the skeleton. The contractions of skeletal muscle are responsible for all voluntary motion. There is no such thing as *rough* muscle.

130. C: *Melatonin* is produced by the pineal gland. One of the primary functions of melatonin is regulation of the circadian cycle, which is the rhythm of sleep and wakefulness. *Insulin* helps regulate the amount of glucose in the blood. Without insulin, the body is unable to convert blood sugar into energy. *Testosterone* is the main hormone produced by the testes; it is responsible for the development of adult male sex characteristics. *Epinephrine*, also

known as adrenaline, performs a number of functions: It quickens and strengthens the heartbeat and dilates the bronchioles. Epinephrine is one of the hormones secreted when the body senses danger.

131. D: Only cells with a membrane around the nucleus are called eukaryotes.

132. C: The two types of cellular transport are active (which requires the cell to invest energy) and passive (which does not require the cell to expend energy).

133. C: There are three states of matter: gases, liquids, and solids.

134. D: An element is a substance that cannot be broken into simpler types of matter.

135. B: Anatomy is the study of the structure and shape of the body.

136. B: It is true that rocks are classified by their formation and the minerals they contain, while minerals are classified by their chemical composition and physical properties. Answer A is incorrect because rocks may contain traces of organic compounds. Answers C and D are incorrect because only minerals can be polymorphs and only rocks contain mineraloids.

137. A: There are four basic tissue types in humans: epithelial, connective, nervous and muscular.

138. A: Aerobic means in the presence of oxygen.

139. A: Chemical composition is not one of the physical properties used to classify minerals. The five major physical properties used to classify minerals are luster, hardness, cleavage, streak, and form. There is a separate classification system based on the chemical composition of minerals.

140. C: Overgrazing and deforestation directly contribute to soil erosion by destroying the natural groundcover that normally prevents soil from being washed and blown away. These activities can ultimately result in desertification, which renders land unsuitable for agriculture.

141. A: Physiology is the study of how parts of the body function.

142. C: On Mohs scale of mineral hardness, talc has the lowest possible score (a one). Diamond is a ten, which is the highest possible score, and gypsum and fluorite have a score of two and four, respectively. Minerals can always scratch minerals that have a Mohs score lower than their own.

143. B: The only purpose of muscles is to produce movement through contraction.

144. D: Weathering causes erosion, which often leads to transportation and the deposition of eroded material. After the eroded material is deposited in a new location, lithification proceeds and the sedimentary cycle begins anew.

145. D: Water is likely to have the shortest residence time in the atmosphere. Water molecules linger in the atmosphere for an estimated 9 days, while their residence time in glaciers may range from 20 to 100 years. Water molecules reside in lakes for approximately 50 to 100 years, and they stay in rivers for two to six months.

146. B: When an earthquake occurs, the "shaking" that is observed is a direct result of seismic waves. Seismic waves are powerful sound waves released when slippage between plates occurs. There are two types of seismic waves: primary, or P-waves, and secondary, or S-waves. P-waves move more quickly than S-waves, and create motion that radiates directly outward from the point of origin. S-waves produce a shearing, or side-to-side, motion.

147. B: An atom with an electrical charge is called an ion.

148. C: When water changes directly from a solid to a gas, skipping the liquid state, it is known as sublimation. It typically occurs when snow or ice is exposed to direct sunlight, and it is possible at unusually low atmospheric pressure points.

149. D: The two types of measurement important in science are quantitative (when a numerical result is used) and qualitative (when descriptions or qualities are reported).

150. D: It is true that the ocean's salinity is usually between 34 and 35 parts per thousand, or 200 parts per million. Oceans comprise about 70.8 percent of the Earth's surface, and the ocean's deepest point is over 10,000 meters below sea level. The Mediterranean is considered a sea, not an ocean.

151. B: Approximately 96.5 percent of seawater is comprised of hydrogen and oxygen. Although seawater does contain sodium, chlorine, magnesium, sulfur, and other dissolved solids, its primary components are the same substances that make up fresh water.

152. A: Circulation is transporting oxygen and other nutrients to the tissues via the cardiovascular system.

153. B: Stratigraphic dating is not a radiometric dating process because it does not consider the radioactive properties of materials to estimate their dates. Instead, it relies on the Law of Superposition to estimate relative ages by comparing the relative depths of materials.

154. D: A solid turns to a liquid by melting, and a liquid turns to a gas by vaporization.

155. A: A fossil that is 37 million years old is an example of an absolute age. Absolute dating, which can be accomplished through the use of radiometric techniques, establishes precise ages for materials, while stratigraphic techniques only produce relative dates. Relative dating can pinpoint approximate ages for rocks and fossils based on clues in the surrounding rock, but it cannot be used to determine absolute age.

156. B: Mass is not the same as weight; rather, mass is the quantity of matter an object has.
157. C: Prokaryotes, or simple cells that lack a nucleus, appeared on Earth approximately 3.8 billion years ago. Eukaryotes, or complex cells, emerged 2 billion years ago, and arthropods developed about 570 million years ago. Amphibians emerged approximately

360 million years ago.

158. B: The first law of classical thermodynamics states that energy can neither be created nor destroyed. The zeroth law is concerned with thermodynamic equilibrium, and the second and third laws discuss entropy.

159. B: The lymphatic system includes the spleen.

160. A: The formula for calculating kinetic energy is ½ mv², where m=mass and v=velocity. Kinetic energy is defined as the energy of an object in motion. Potential energy, or stored energy, is measured using the formula mgh, where m=mass, g=gravity, and h=height.

Practice Test #2

Practice Questions

Verbal Review

1. Administration of the indicated drug will *ameliorate* the patient's condition.
Ameliorate means:
    a. improve
    b. worsen
    c. intensify
    d. cure

2. The hospital staff listened to the chief of staff's *fervent* speech regarding proposed changes at the facility.
Fervent means:
    a. enthusiastic
    b. dispassionate
    c. emotional
    d. lengthy

3. Some of the hospital's computer equipment is *outmoded*.
Outmoded means:
    a. inoperable
    b. refurbished
    c. worn-out
    d. obsolete

4. The accident victim's arm is *saturated in* blood.
Saturated means:
    a. caked
    b. wet
    c. inundated
    d. steeped

5. Mark's concerned daughter brought him into the emergency room, and it was found that he had *feigned* a heart attack.
Feigned means:
    a. undergone
    b. experienced
    c. affected
    d. concealed

6. The medical center's chief operating officer is an *exponent* of patient's rights.
Exponent means:
    a. advocate
    b. opponent
    c. adherent
    d. critic

7. A report has been filed regarding the pharmaceutical company's *delusive* practices.
Delusive means:
    a. lauded
    b. aboveboard
    c. dishonest
    d. deceptive

8. The patient's body strength *languished* over the course of her stay at the hospital.
Languished means:
    a. recovered
    b. weakened
    c. broke down
    d. stabilized

9. Allowing most visitors into the operating room is *incongruous*.
Incongruous means:
    a. forbidden
    b. unacceptable
    c. inappropriate
    d. befitting

10. The head nurse was *contrite* about the order she had given.
Contrite means:
    a. unapologetic
    b. sorry
    c. unyielding
    d. empowered

11. The patient's voice was quite *husky*.
Husky means:
    a. mellow
    b. abrasive
    c. strained
    d. hoarse

12. The physical therapist *demurred* regarding the doctor's suggested course of therapy.
Demurred means:
    a. objected
    b. concurred
    c. complied with
    d. agonized

13. The hospital auditorium is used for lectures and other events because it is *capacious*.
Capacious means:
    a. grand
    b. remodeled
    c. spacious
    d. retrofitted

14. The head nurse *harbors* a grudge against the supervising physician.
Harbors means:
    a. maintains
    b. renounces
    c. picks
    d. bears

15. Lydia tried every possible way to *circumvent* her doctor's orders.
Circumvent means:
    a. follow
    b. acquiesce to
    c. skirt
    d. eschew

16. In hospital laboratories, compliance with federal regulations regarding handling of blood is *mandatory*.
Mandatory means:
    a. obligatory
    b. essential
    c. enforced
    d. discretionary

17. The doctor was sued because he *maligned* his patient.
Maligned means:
    a. hit
    b. slandered
    c. debased
    d. assaulted

18. The storage room was quite *unkempt*.
Unkempt means:
    a. dingy
    b. organized
    c. clean
    d. messy

19. The patient was affected deeply by the *sardonic* remarks of her son.
Sardonic means:
    a. heartfelt
    b. sarcastic
    c. harsh
    d. genial

20. During a fire alarm, everyone should proceed to the *egress.*
Egress means:
    a. hallway
    b. exit
    c. shelter
    d. outdoors

21. There is *parity* between the excellences of care at the two hospitals.
Parity means:
    a. inequality
    b. similarity
    c. equivalence
    d. competition

22. The nursing assistant's manner *estranges* her patients.
Estranges means:
    a. endears
    b. alienates
    c. antagonizes
    d. encourages

23. Amelia was taken aback by her supervisor's *gratuitous* remarks.
Gratuitous means:
    a. hateful
    b. excessive
    c. irrelevant
    d. unnecessary

24. The patient in room 201 has a *voracious* appetite.
Voracious means:
    a. minimal
    b. gluttonous
    c. hearty
    d. bland

25. The exercise involves moving *laterally* on the machine.
Laterally means:
    a. sideways
    b. forward
    c. backward
    d. upward

26. The leukemia patient is quite *dauntless* in his outlook regarding his treatment regimen.
Dauntless means:
    a. fearful
    b. brave
    c. overconfident
    d. disconsolate

27. The doctor looked *askance* at the patient's claim of compliance with his orders.
Askance means:
    a. encouragingly
    b. contemptuously
    c. incredulously
    d. distrustfully

28. Ronald's tibia fracture has not healed *hitherto*.
Hitherto means:
    a. properly
    b. thus far
    c. completely
    d. sufficiently

29. The nursing staff looks to Dr. Waller for his *sage* advice.
Sag" means:
    a. wise
    b. astute
    c. vast
    d. logical

30. Chemotherapy given to terminally ill patients is used to *mitigate* their suffering.
Mitigate means:
    a. lessen
    b. disguise
    c. help
    d. rectify

31. The nurse was quite *forthright* in her conversations with the patient.
Forthright means:
    a. frank
    b. evasive
    c. animated
    d. reticent

32. Elisabeth visited her sister in the hospital every day despite the latter's *dyspeptic* behavior. *Dyspeptic* means:
    a. sullen
    b. erratic
    c. comatose
    d. ill-tempered

33. The administrator spoke with *vehemence* about the proposed merger.
Vehemence means:
    a. intensity
    b. passion
    c. duplicity
    d. ardor

34. The *unflappable* therapist ignored the intruding visitors.
Unflappable means:
   a. unflinching
   b. imperturbable
   c. proficient
   d. diligent

35. Mammography is a *benchmark* for diagnosis of breast cancer.
Benchmark means:
   a. test
   b. pinnacle
   c. standard
   d. method

Questions 36 – 41 pertain to the following passage:

Peanut allergy is the most prevalent food allergy in the United States, affecting around one and a half million people, and it is potentially on the rise in children in the United States. While thought to be the most common cause of food-related death, deaths from food allergies are very rare. The allergy typically begins at a very young age and remains present for life for most people. Approximately one-fifth to one-quarter of children with a peanut allergy, however, outgrow it. Treatment involves careful avoidance of peanuts or any food that may contain peanut pieces or oils. For some sufferers, exposure to even the smallest amount of peanut product can trigger a serious reaction.

Symptoms of peanut allergy can include skin reactions, itching around the mouth, digestive problems, shortness of breath, and runny or stuffy nose. The most severe peanut allergies can result in anaphylaxis, which requires immediate treatment with epinephrine. Up to one-third of people with peanut allergies have severe reactions. Without treatment, anaphylactic shock can result in death due to obstruction of the airway, or heart failure. Signs of anaphylaxis include constriction of airways and difficulty breathing, shock, a rapid pulse, and dizziness or lightheadedness.

As of yet, there is no treatment to prevent or cure allergic reactions to peanuts. In May of 2008, however, Duke University Medical Center food allergy experts announced that they expect to offer a treatment for peanut allergies within five years.

Scientists do not know for sure why peanut proteins induce allergic reactions, nor do they know why some people develop peanut allergies while others do not. There is a strong genetic component to allergies: if one of a child's parents has an allergy, the child has an almost 50% chance of developing an allergy. If both parents have an allergy, the odds increase to about 70%.

Someone suffering from a peanut allergy needs to be cautious about the foods he or she eats and the products he or she puts on his or her skin. Common foods that should be checked for peanut content are ground nuts, cereals, granola, grain breads, energy bars, and salad dressings. Store prepared cookies, pastries, and frozen desserts like ice cream can also contain peanuts. Additionally, many cuisines use peanuts in cooking – watch

- 51 -

for peanut content in African, Chinese, Indonesian, Mexican, Thai, and Vietnamese dishes.

Parents of children with peanut allergies should notify key people (child care providers, school personnel, etc.) that their child has a peanut allergy, explain peanut allergy symptoms to them, make sure that the child's epinephrine auto injector is always available, write an action plan of care for their child when he or she has an allergic reaction to peanuts, have their child wear a medical alert bracelet or necklace, and discourage their child from sharing foods.

36. According to the passage, approximately what percentage of people with peanut allergies have severe reactions?
    a. Up to 11%
    b. Up to 22%
    c. Up to 33%
    d. Up to 44%

37. By what date do Duke University allergy experts expect to offer a treatment for peanut allergies?
    a. 2008
    b. 2009
    c. 2010
    d. 2013

38. Which of the following is not a type of cuisine the passage suggests often contains peanuts?
    a. African
    b. Italian
    c. Vietnamese
    d. Mexican

39. Which allergy does the article state is thought to be the most common cause of food-related death?
    a. Peanut
    b. Tree nut
    c. Bee sting
    d. Poison oak

40. It can be inferred from the passage that children with peanut allergies should be discouraged from sharing food because:
    a. Peanut allergies can be contagious.
    b. People suffering from peanut allergies are more susceptible to bad hygiene.
    c. Many foods contain peanut content and it is important to be very careful when you don't know what you're eating.
    d. Scientists don't know why some people develop peanut allergies.

41. Which of the following does the passage not state is a sign of anaphylaxis?
   a. constriction of airways
   b. shock
   c. a rapid pulse
   d. running or stuffy nose

Questions 42 – 45 pertain to the following passage:

It is most likely that you have never had diphtheria. You probably don't even know anyone who has suffered from this disease. In fact, you may not even know what diphtheria is. Similarly, diseases like whooping cough, measles, mumps, and rubella may all be unfamiliar to you. In the nineteenth and early twentieth centuries, these illnesses struck hundreds of thousands of people in the United States each year, mostly children, and tens of thousands of people died. The names of these diseases were frightening household words. Today, they are all but forgotten. That change happened largely because of vaccines.

You probably have been vaccinated against diphtheria. You may even have been exposed to the bacterium that causes it, but the vaccine prepared your body to fight off the disease so quickly that you were unaware of the infection. Vaccines take advantage of your body's natural ability to learn how to combat many disease-causing germs, or microbes. What's more, your body remembers how to protect itself from the microbes it has encountered before. Collectively, the parts of your body that remember and repel microbes are called the immune system. Without the proper functioning of the immune system, the simplest illness—even the common cold—could quickly turn deadly.

On average, your immune system needs more than a week to learn how to fight off an unfamiliar microbe. Sometimes, that isn't enough time. Strong microbes can spread through your body faster than the immune system can fend them off. Your body often gains the upper hand after a few weeks, but in the meantime you are sick. Certain microbes are so virulent that they can overwhelm or escape your natural defenses. In those situations, vaccines can make all the difference.

Traditional vaccines contain either parts of microbes or whole microbes that have been altered so that they don't cause disease. When your immune system confronts these harmless versions of the germs, it quickly clears them from your body. In other words, vaccines trick your immune system in order to teach your body important lessons about how to defeat its opponents.

42. What is the main idea of the passage?
   a. The nineteenth and early twentieth centuries were a dark period for medicine.
   b. You have probably never had diphtheria.
   c. Traditional vaccines contain altered microbes.
   d. Vaccines help the immune system function properly.

43. Which statement is *not* a detail from the passage?
   a. Vaccines contain microbe parts or altered microbes.
   b. The immune system typically needs a week to learn how to fight a new disease.
   c. The symptoms of disease do not emerge until the body has learned how to fight the microbe.
   d. A hundred years ago, children were at the greatest risk of dying from now-treatable diseases.

44. What is the meaning of the word *virulent* as it is used in the third paragraph?
   a. tiny
   b. malicious
   c. contagious
   d. annoying

45. What is the author's primary purpose in writing the essay?
   a. to entertain
   b. to persuade
   c. to inform
   d. to analyze

Questions 46 – 49 pertain to the following passage:

Among the Atkins, South Beach and other diets people embark upon for health and weight loss is the so-called Paleolithic Diet in which adherents eat what they believe to be a diet similar to that consumed by humans during the Paleolithic era. The diet consists of food that can be hunted or gathered: primarily of meat, fish, vegetables, fruits, roots, and nuts. It does not allow for grains, legumes, dairy, salt, refined sugars or processed oils. The idea behind the diet is that humans are genetically adapted to the diet of our Paleolithic forebears. Some studies support the idea of positive health outcomes from such a diet.

46. Which of the following does the passage not give as the name of a diet?
   a. South Beach
   b. Hunter Gatherer
   c. Paleolithic
   d. Atkins

47. Which of the following is not permitted on the Paleolithic Diet?
   a. meat
   b. dairy
   c. vegetables
   d. nuts

48. What does the passage say is the idea behind the diet?
   a. That humans are genetically adapted to the diet of our Paleolithic forebears
   b. That it increases health
   c. That it supports weight loss
   d. That it consists of food that can be hunted or gathered

49. Which of the following does the passage suggest is true?
    a. No studies support the claim that the Paleolithic Diet promotes health
    b. Some studies support the claim that the Paleolithic Diet promotes health
    c. All studies support the claim that the Paleolithic Diet promotes health
    d. No studies have been done on whether the Paleolithic Diet promotes health

Use the following information to answer questions 50 -54:
    Directions: For the relief of headaches. Take one pill every 4 to 6 hours, not exceeding 4 in a 24-hour period. If stomach upset occurs, take with food. If pain persists more than 24 hours, contact a physician.

50. The medication should be taken:
    a. 6 times a day
    b. every thirty minutes
    c. on an empty stomach
    d. to treat a headache

51. Upset means
    a. angry
    b. annoyed
    c. physical disorder
    d. confusion

52. If someone follows the directions, what is the maximum number of pills he or she should have taken before he or she could first contact a physician?
    a. 2
    b. 3
    c. 4
    d. 6

53. Persists means
    a. tries
    b. continues
    c. hurts
    d. worsens

54. What is the maximum number of pills, including the first one, that could be taken in the 12 hours upon starting to use this medication?
    a. 2
    b. 3
    c. 4
    d. 5

Questions 55- 60 pertain to the following information:
Tips for Eating Calcium Rich Foods
    Include milk as a beverage at meals. Choose fat-free or low-fat milk. If you usually drink whole milk, switch gradually to fat-free milk to lower saturated fat and calories. Try reduced fat (2%), then low-fat (1%), and finally fat-free (skim).

- 55 -

If you drink cappuccinos or lattes—ask for them with fat-free (skim) milk.
Add fat-free or low-fat milk instead of water to oatmeal and hot cereals
Use fat-free or low-fat milk when making condensed cream soups (such as cream of tomato).
Have fat-free or low-fat yogurt as a snack.
Make a dip for fruits or vegetables from yogurt.
Make fruit-yogurt smoothies in the blender.
For dessert, make chocolate or butterscotch pudding with fat-free or low-fat milk.
Top cut-up fruit with flavored yogurt for a quick dessert.
Top casseroles, soups, stews, or vegetables with shredded low-fat cheese.
Top a baked potato with fat-free or low-fat yogurt.

For those who choose not to consume milk products:
If you avoid milk because of lactose intolerance, the most reliable way to get the health benefits of milk is to choose lactose-free alternatives within the milk group, such as cheese, yogurt, or lactose-free milk, or to consume the enzyme lactase before consuming milk products.
Calcium choices for those who do not consume milk products include:
- Calcium fortified juices, cereals, breads, soy beverages, or rice beverages
- Canned fish (sardines, salmon with bones) soybeans and other soy products, some other dried beans, and some leafy greens.

55. According to the passage, how can you lower saturated fat and calories in your diet?
    a. Add fat-free milk to oatmeal instead of water.
    b. Switch to fat-free milk.
    c. Drink calcium-fortified juice.
    d. Make yogurt dip.

56. What device does the author use to organize the passage?
    a. headings
    b. captions
    c. diagrams
    d. labels

57. How much fat does reduced fat milk contain?
    a. 0 percent
    b. 1 percent
    c. 2 percent
    d. 3 percent

58. Which of the following is true about calcium rich foods?
    I. Canned salmon with bones contains calcium.
    II. Cheese is a lactose-free food.
    III. Condensed soup made with water is a calcium rich food.
   a. I only
   b. I and II only
   c. II and III only
   d. III only

59. What information should the author include to help clarify information in the passage?
   a. The fat content of yogurt.
   b. How much calcium is in fortified juice.
   c. Which leafy greens contain calcium.
   d. The definition of lactose intolerance.

60. The style of this passage is most like that found in a(n)
   a. tourist guidebook.
   b. friendly letter.
   c. encyclopedia.
   d. health textbook.

61. 14,634
   + 7,377

   a. 21,901
   b. 21,911
   c. 22,011
   d. 22,901

62.   9,645
   - 6,132

   a. 2,513
   b. 2,517
   c. 3,412
   d. 3,513

63. What is the value of r in the following equation?
   $$29 + r = 420$$
   a. $r = 29/420$
   b. $r = 420/29$
   c. $r = 391$
   d. $r = 449$

64.   893
   x   64

   a. 54,142
   b. 56,822
   c. 56,920
   d. 57,152

65.   649
   x   7

   a. 4,473
   b. 4,483
   c. 4,543
   d. 4,573

66. Find the area of the rectangle.

5ft

7 ft

    a. 5 ft²
    b. 12 ft²
    c. 24 ft²
    d. 35 ft²

67. $9\overline{)863}$
    a. 89 R2
    b. 93 R2
    c. 95 R8
    d. 96 R8

68. $97\overline{)29294}$
    a. 302
    b. 322
    c. 3002
    d. 3022

69. If 35% of a paycheck was deducted for taxes and 4% for insurance, what is the total percent taken out of the paycheck?
    a. 20%
    b. 31%
    c. 39%
    d. 42%

70. 0.28 x 0.17
    a. 0.2260
    b. 0.4760
    c. 0.0226
    d. 0.0476

71. 0.8/1.6 is equal to
    a. 0.02
    b. 0.05
    c. 0.2
    d. 0.5

72. Which of the following choices expresses 5/8 as a percent?
 a. 40%
 b. 58%
 c. 62.5%
 d. 65%

73. Round off to the nearest hundredth: 0.1673
 a. 0.16
 b. 0.166
 c. 0.167
 d. 0.17

74. What is the equivalent decimal number for five hundred twelve thousandths?
 a. 0.512
 b. 0.0512
 c. 5120.
 d. 0.00512

75. The scientific notation for a red blood cell is approximately 7.4×10^{-4} centimeters in diameter. What is that amount in standard form?
 a. 0.00074
 b. 0.0074
 c. 7.40000
 d. 296

76. $3/5 \div 1/2$
 a. 1 1/5
 b. 3/10
 c. 1 7/10
 d. 4/5

77. Which of the following is correct?
 a. 4/7 = 12/21
 b. 3/4 = 12/20
 c. 5/8 = 15/32
 d. 7/9 = 28/35

78. Find N for the following:
$n/7 = 18/21$
 a. 3
 b. 4
 c. 5
 d. 6

79. A woman wants to stack two small bookcases beneath a window that is 26½ inches from the floor. The larger bookcase is 14½ inches tall. The other bookcase is 8¾ inches tall. How tall with the two bookcases be when they are stacked together?

    a. 12 inches tall
    b. 23¼ inches tall
    c. 35¼ inches tall
    d. 41 inches tall

80. Express 68/7 as a mixed fraction.

    a. 9 5/7
    b. 8 4/7
    c. 9 3/7
    d. 8 6/7

81. 3=(?%) of 60

    a. 5
    b. 9
    c. 15
    d. 20

82. 1 is what percent of 25?

    a. 1%
    b. 2%
    c. 3%
    d. 4%

83. Solve for y in the following equation if $x = -3$

$y = x + 5$

    a. $y = -2$
    b. $y = 2$
    c. $y = 3$
    d. $y = 8$

84. $1/3 = (?)\% \times 5/6$

    a. 10
    b. 20
    c. 30
    d. 40

85. 5/8 as a decimal

    a. .37
    b. .62
    c. .375
    d. .625

86. 0.023 as a percentage
    a. 23%
    b. 2.3%
    c. .23%
    d. .023%

87. It costs $2.50 to make a 15 minute phone call. At the same rate, how much will it cost to make a phone call that lasts 12 minutes?
    a. $1.50
    b. $1.75
    c. $2.00
    d. $2.25

88. 12 is 25% of x
    a. 28
    b. 36
    c. 40
    d. 48

89. 32% of x = 96
    a. 208
    b. 250
    c. 280
    d. 300

90. $4ax^2 - 8ax^2$
    a. $4ax^2$
    b. $-4ax^2$
    c. $12ax^2$
    d. $-12ax^2$

91. Put the following integers in order from greatest to least:
-52, 16, -12, 14, 8, -5, 0
    a. -52, 16, -12, 14, 8, -5, 0
    b. 0, -5, 8, -12, 14, 16, -52
    c. 0, -5, -12, -52, 8, 14, 16
    d. 16, 14, 8, 0, -5, -12, -52

92. $4(x + 2) - 3 + 3(x + 5)$
    a. $x + 23$
    b. $7x + 20$
    c. $4x + 3$
    d. $7x + 9$

93. $4x - 5 = 23$
    a. $x = 4$
    b. $x = 5$
    c. $x = 6$
    d. $x = 7$

94. $2(r + 4) + 8 = (r + 3)4$
    a. $r = -2$
    b. $r = 2$
    c. $r = -4$
    d. $r = 4$

95. If number x is subtracted from 27, the result is -5. What is number x?
    a. 22
    b. 25
    c. 32
    d. 35

96. Which of the following is true?
    a. -(-(-4)) is greater than -3
    b. -(-7) is greater than 17 minus 10
    c. -4 is greater than the absolute value of -4
    d. -10 is greater than -(-(-15))

97. How many cubic inches are in a box 10" wide, 3" deep and 14" long?
    a. 420
    b. 4200
    c. 210
    d. 2100

98. Solve the equation: $2^3 + (4 + 1)$.
    a. 9
    b. 13
    c. 15
    d. 21

99. What does $4x - 1/2y$ equal if $x = 9$ and $y = 6$
    a. 36
    b. 33
    c. 30
    d. 26

100. Which algebraic expression best represents the following statement: the number of books Brian read over the summer (B) is 2 less than 3 times the number of books his brother Adam read over the summer (A)?
    a. $B = 3A - 2$
    b. $B = 3A + 2$
    c. $A = 3B - 2$
    d. $A = 3B + 2$

101. The adrenal glands are part of the
    a. immune system.
    b. endocrine system.
    c. emphatic system.
    d. respiratory system.

102. Which of the following is exchanged between two or more atoms that undergo ionic bonding?
    a. neutrons
    b. transitory electrons
    c. valence electrons
    d. electrical charges

103. Which of the following statements is *not* true of most metals?
    a. They are good conductors of heat.
    b. They are gases at room temperature.
    c. They are ductile.
    d. They make up the majority of elements on the periodic table.

104. What is most likely the pH of a solution containing many hydroxide ions (OH⁻) and few hydrogen ions (H⁺)?
    a. 2
    b. 6
    c. 7
    d. 9

105. Which of the following cannot be found on the periodic table?
    a. bromine
    b. magnesium oxide
    c. phosphorous
    d. chlorine

106. A cyclist is riding over a hill. At what point is his potential energy greatest?
    a. at the base of the hill
    b. halfway up the hill
    c. at the very top of the hill
    d. on the way down the hill

107. Which of the following correctly describes the trait Ll, if "L" represents tallness and "l" represents shortness?
    a. heterozygous genotype and tall phenotype
    b. heterozygous phenotype and tall genotype
    c. homozygous genotype and short phenotype
    d. homozygous phenotype and short genotype

108. What law describes the electric force between two charged particles?
   a. Ohm's law
   b. Coulomb's law
   c. The Doppler effect
   d. Kirchhoff's current law

109. What is the name of the organelle that organizes protein synthesis?
   a. mitochondrion
   b. nucleus
   c. ribosome
   d. vacuole

110. What is the mass (in grams) of 1.0 mol oxygen gas?
   a. 12 g
   b. 16 g
   c. 28 g
   d. 32 g

111. How much air does an adult inhale in an average breath?
   a. 500 mL
   b. 750 mL
   c. 1000 mL
   d. 1250 mL

112. During which phase is the chromosome number reduced from diploid to haploid?
   a. S phase
   b. interphase
   c. mitosis
   d. meiosis I

113. Which kind of radiation has no charge?
   a. beta
   b. alpha
   c. delta
   d. gamma

114. Which force motivates filtration in the kidneys?
   a. osmosis
   b. smooth muscle contraction
   c. peristalsis
   d. blood pressure

115. Which of the following forms of water is the densest?
   a. liquid
   b. steam
   c. ice
   d. All forms of water have the same density.

116. What is the name of the state in which forward and reverse chemical reactions are occurring at the same rate?
   a. equilibrium
   b. constancy
   c. stability
   d. toxicity

117. Which of the following hormones decreases the concentration of blood glucose?
   a. insulin
   b. glucagon
   c. growth hormone
   d. glucocorticoids

118. What is the longest phase in the life of a cell?
   a. prophase
   b. interphase
   c. anaphase
   d. metaphase

119. What is 119°K in degrees Celsius?
   a. 32°C
   b. –154°C
   c. 154°C
   d. –32°C

120. How much of a female's blood volume is composed of red blood cells?
   a. 10%
   b. 25%
   c. 40%
   d. 70%

121. Which of the following is *not* found within a bacterial cell?
   a. mitochondria
   b. DNA
   c. vesicles
   d. ribosome

122. What is the SI unit of energy?
   a. ohm
   b. joule
   c. henry
   d. newton

123. Which type of cholesterol is considered to be the best for health?
   a. LDL
   b. HDL
   c. VLDL
   d. VHDL

124. Which of the following structures is *not* involved in translation?
a. tRNA
b. mRNA
c. ribosome
d. DNA

125. What is the name of the device that separates gaseous ions by their mass-to-charge ratio?
a. mass spectrometer
b. interferometer
c. magnetometer
d. capacitance meter

126. Where does gas exchange occur in the human body?
a. alveoli
b. bronchi
c. larynx
d. pharynx

127. How many different types of nucleotides are there in DNA?
a. one
b. two
c. four
d. eight

128. What are van der Waals forces?
a. the weak forces of attraction between two molecules
b. the strong forces of attraction between two molecules
c. hydrogen bonds
d. conjugal bonds

129. What is the name of the process in the lungs by which oxygen is transported from the air to the blood?
a. osmosis
b. diffusion
c. dissipation
d. reverse osmosis

130. Which part of aerobic respiration uses oxygen?
a. osmosis
b. Krebs cycle
c. glycolysis
d. electron transport system

131. Which of the following is the correct formula for converting Fahrenheit to Celsius?
a. 5/9 (F - 32)
b. 9/5 (F - 32)
c. 5/9 (F + 32)
d. None of the above

132. A calorimeter is used to measure changes in:
    a. Heat.
    b. Mass.
    c. Weight.
    d. Volume.

133. Which of the following is a vector quantity?
    a. Distance
    b. Speed
    c. Velocity
    d. Time

134. According to the Dana classification system, minerals that contain the anion SO_4^{2-} are part of which chemical class?
    a. Sulfate
    b. Sulfite
    c. Halide
    d. Phosphate

135. Which of the following statements about energy is true?
    a. Mechanical energy is always conserved in an isolated system.
    b. Total energy is always conserved in an isolated system.
    c. Energy is never created or destroyed.
    d. You can determine the mechanical energy of an object by using the equation $E = mc^2$

136. Physical weathering of rocks can be caused by all of the following EXCEPT:
    a. The freezing and thawing of water on the surface of rocks.
    b. Changes in temperature.
    c. Oxidation.
    d. Changes in pressure due to the removal of overlying rocks.

137. Ultrasound imaging, which is used for various medical procedures, including imaging pregnant women, is based on which of the following principles.
    a. Doppler effect.
    b. Echolocation
    c. Infrasonic.
    d. Resonance.

138. Which of the following statements is true of a closed thermodynamic system?
    a. It cannot exchange heat, work, or matter with its surrounding environment.
    b. It can exchange heat and work, but not matter, with its surrounding environment.
    c. It can exchange heat, but not work or matter, with its surrounding environment.
    d. It can exchange matter, but not heat or work, with its surrounding environment.

139. An object with a net charge is brought into the vicinity of an object with a net charge of zero coulombs. Which statement describes the electrostatic force between the two objects?
a. It is a repulsive force.
b. It is an attractive force.
c. There is no force.
d. It is a perpendicular force.

140. Which of the following is the correct definition of a conductor?
a. A metal wire in an electrical circuit.
b. A material that contains moveable electric charges.
c. A material that is not a semiconductor or insulator.
d. Any device that allows electricity to flow.

141. All of the following are examples of metamorphic rocks EXCEPT:
a. Granite.
b. Quartzite.
c. Slate.
d. Marble.

142. Which of the following devices changes chemical energy into electrical energy?
a. battery
b. closed electric circuit
c. generator
d. transformer

143. Which of the following statements explains what causes a rainbow?
a. The components of sunlight strike water droplets at different angles.
b. Water molecules produce an emission spectrum when sunlight strikes them.
c. The speed of light in water depends on its wavelength.
d. There is total internal reflection for certain wavelengths of sunlight.

144. The state of matter in which atoms have the strongest bond is:
a. Plasma.
b. Liquid.
c. Solid.
d. Gas.

145. Which of the following statements about isotopes of an element is true?
a. They have the same number of nucleons.
b. They have the same number of neutrons, but different numbers of protons.
c. They have the same number of protons, but different numbers of neutrons.
d. They have a different number of electrons.

146. A gas at constant volume is cooled. Which statement about the gas must be true?
a. The kinetic energy of the gas molecules has decreased.
b. The gas has condensed to a liquid.
c. The weight of the gas has decreased.
d. The density of the gas has increased.

147. Chemical compounds are formed when:
    a. Valence electrons from atoms of two different elements are shared or transferred.
    b. Valence electrons from multiple atoms of a single element are shared or transferred.
    c. The nuclei of two atoms are joined together.
    d. The nucleus of an atom is split.

148. One mole of oxygen gas and two moles of hydrogen are combined in a sealed container at STP. Which of the following statements is true?
    a. The mass of hydrogen gas is greater than the mass of oxygen.
    b. The volume of hydrogen is greater than the volume of oxygen.
    c. The hydrogen and oxygen will react to produce 2 mol of water.
    d. The partial pressure of hydrogen is greater than the partial pressure of oxygen.

149. The process that causes lithospheric plates to move over the surface of the mantle is called:
    a. Conduction.
    b. Convection.
    c. Tension.
    d. Subduction.

150. Which of the following statements about radioactive decay is true?
    a. The sum of the mass of the daughter particles is less than that of the parent nucleus
    b. The sum of the mass of the daughter particles is greater than that of the parent nucleus
    c. The sum of the mass of the daughter particles is equal to that of the parent nucleus
    d. The sum of the mass of the daughter particles cannot be accurately measured

151. Adding a catalyst to a reaction will do which of the following to that reaction:
    a. Shift the reaction equilibrium towards the products
    b. Increase the temperature of the reaction
    c. Decrease the energy of activation for the reaction
    d. Increase the purity of the reaction products

152. Proteins are made up of which of the following repeating subunits?
    a. Sugars
    b. Triglycerides
    c. Amino acids
    d. Nucleic acids

153. Galena, pyrite, and magnetite are examples of minerals with which of the following types of luster?
    a. Pearly
    b. Greasy
    c. Adamantine
    d. Metallic

154. The precision of a number of data points refers to:
    a. How accurate the data is
    b. How many errors the data contains
    c. How close the data points are to the mean of the data
    d. How close the actual data is to the predicted result

155. The density of a material refers to:
    a. Mass per volume
    b. Mass per mole
    c. Molecular weight per volume
    d. Moles per volume

156. Water's specific heat capacity is second only to that of ammonia. This means that:
    a. Water vaporizes at a higher temperature than ammonia.
    b. It takes more energy to increase the temperature of ammonia than it does to increase the temperature of water.
    c. Water is always denser than ammonia.
    d. Water is only denser than ammonia at higher temperatures.

157. Which of the following statements is NOT true of electrons?
    a. They comprise only a tiny fraction of an atom's mass.
    b. They are arranged in levels, and usually occupy the lowest energy level possible.
    c. They are negatively charged.
    d. They have a substructure that includes a nucleus.

158. Which statement about the impact of chemistry on society is not true?
    a. Fluoridation of water has had no effect on the rate of cavities as compared to unfluoridated water
    b. Chemical fertilizers have tremendously increased food production per acre in the U.S.
    c. Chemistry played a central role in the development of nuclear weapons
    d. Use of catalytic converters in automobiles has greatly reduced acid rain producing exhaust products

159. In geochronology, which of the following is the longest time period?
    a. An epoch
    b. An era
    c. An eon
    d. An age

160. The atomic number of an element is defined by:
    a. The total number of protons and electrons it contains.
    b. The total number of electrons it contains.
    c. The total number of protons it contains.
    d. The total number of neutrons it contains.

Answer Key and Explanations

Verbal Review

1. A: *Improve* is a synonym for *ameliorate*, both of which mean "to make better." *Intensify* is similar, but this word implies an effort greater in degree or measurement. *Worsen* is the antonym meaning, "to become worse or less in value." Cure could fit into this sentence, as it means, "to effect recovery from," but does not relate directly to *ameliorate*.

2. C: *Emotional* is the only true synonym for *fervent*, which means "showing great depth of feeling or passionate enthusiasm." Therefore, *dispassionate*, which means "uninfluenced by emotion or personal feelings," is an antonym. *Enthusiastic* implies urgency of desire or interest, and this word is synonymous with *eager*. *Lengthy* (or long) is unrelated to the term *fervent*.

3. D: *Obsolete* and *outmoded* are synonyms, both connoting "having surpassed its time of use or usefulness." *Worn-out* is related, but this word suggests something is "damaged or weakened through prolonged use." In this context, *inoperable* describes something "not workable or practical," making it a related word as well. *Refurbished* means, "restored to good repair," and is a near antonym.

4. B: *Wet* and *saturated* are synonyms, both meaning "covered with, containing, or penetrated with liquid." Inundated is a related term in this case meaning, "flooded," but this word can also mean "overwhelmed." Similarly, *steeped* means, "soaked or immersed in liquid." In this sentence, *caked* would mean, "forming a crust."

5. C: *Affected* is the synonym for *feigned* because in this instance both words mean, "presenting a false appearance of." *Concealed* is a somewhat related term signifying that something is "hidden." The other choices fit into the sentence and are synonyms for each other; as verbs, *undergone* and *experienced* both mean, "having come to knowledge of something by living through it."

6. A: An *exponent* is an *advocate*, someone who actively promotes or favors a cause. *Adherent* is a somewhat related term meaning, "follower, someone who follows the opinions or teachings of others." *Opponent* is an antonym signifying, "one who takes an opposing position." *Critic* is a near antonym, which in this sentence would mean "fault-finder."

7. D: *Deceptive* and *delusive* are synonyms meaning, "tending or possessing power to deceive". *Dishonest* is a stronger related word that means, "meant to deceive, swindle or trick." *Aboveboard* is an antonym connoting that something is "honest, legal, and lacking in deception." *Lauded* could be inserted in this sentence, but it is a completely unrelated term meaning, "highly praised."

8. B: *Languished* is a synonym for one of the meanings of weakened, which is "lost bodily strength or vigor." In this case, *broke down* is a related expression that means, "having

decayed or failed." In this sentence, *recovered* is a near antonym meaning, "having regained a former, normal, or healthy and strong state." Stabilized, though unrelated, could be inserted in this sentence to mean, "having become constant."

9. C: *Inappropriate* is a synonym for *incongruous*, which in this context means "not appropriate for the occasion or situation." Incongruous can also mean "inconsistent." Two of the other words are related terms: (1) *forbidden*, which means "not permitted," and (2) *unacceptable*, which means "falling short of a standard." *Befitting* is an antonym defined as "appropriate for."

10. B: Contrite has two possible definitions, which are either "sorry" or "guilty," and therefore B is the correct answer of choices presented. *Unapologetic* is an antonym for the first sense meaning, "not feeling sorrow for a wrong one has done." The other choices could be used in the sentence but are unrelated. *Unyielding* can mean either "stubborn" or "inflexible," and empowered can mean either "given authority" or "made more assertive or confident."

11. D: *Hoarse* is the only true synonym for *husky*, both meaning "harsh and dry sounding." Two of the answers are related terms: (1) *abrasive*, which is defined as "harsh in *manner*" (also "using friction"), and (2) *strained*, which in this context means "not natural or spontaneous." *Mellow* is an antonym meaning "lyrical" or "gentle."

12. A: *Demurred*, the form of "demur" used here, is a verb, and therefore it is synonymous with *objected*. Both verbs here would mean, "presented a contrary opinion or argument." *Concurred* is almost the opposite, meaning, "had the same opinion as." *Complied* is defined as "obeyed or conformed to." In this context, *agonized* means, "spent time worrying before making a decision."

13. C: *Capacious* and *spacious* both mean "more than adequate in terms of capacity." *Grand* has several meanings, but in this sentence the applicable meaning is "large and impressive in size or grandeur." The other words, although unrelated terms, could be inserted. *Remodeled* means "renovated," and *retrofitted* means "modified or installed with new parts."

14. D: As a verb, *harbor* has several meanings, but in this context *harbors* is synonymous with *bears*. Here both mean, "keeps in one's heart or mind." *Maintains* is a related word; the definition most applicable here is "upholds or continues to declare." *Renounces* is a near antonym, and in this sentence would mean, "rejects or goes back on." In this context, *picks* would mean, "starts a fight or argument with."

15. C: *Skirt* is the only true synonym for *circumvent*, which in this instance means, "to avoid having to comply with, especially using cleverness." *Eschew* is a related word meaning "to abstain from." *Follow* is an antonym; of the word's numerous meanings, the closest in this context would be "to obey." The expression *acquiesce to* would almost be an antonym meaning, "to comply in a passive manner."

16. A: *Obligatory* is synonymous with *mandatory*, which means "required by or as if by law." The Occupational Safety and Health Administration (OSHA) does in fact issue mandatory standards regarding handling of blood. Two of the terms presented are related words: (1) *essential*, which here would signify "impossible to do without," and (2) *enforced*, which

means "carried out effectively." *Discretionary* is a near antonym meaning "optional or subject to freedom of choice."

17. B: The verbs *malign* and *slander* both mean "to make false and damaging statements about," actions for which one can be sued. *Debased* is a related term meaning, "reduced someone in status or significance." A professional could be sued for committing the other options listed as well. In this sentence, *hit* would mean, "to deliver a blow to forcefully" which could be considered "battery," a criminal offense defined as "the unlawful use of force on someone." In this context, *assault* most likely would mean, "an unlawful threat of bodily harm."

18. D: *Unkempt* can mean "sloppy," but in this case, it is synonymous with *messy*. The definition of both terms applicable here is "lacking in order, neatness, and perhaps cleanliness." *Dingy* is a related term signifying that something is "dirty." *Organized* is the opposite of *unkempt*, meaning "following a systematic pattern or method," and *clean* or "free from dirt" is a near antonym.

19. B: *Sarcastic* is a synonym for *sardonic*, defined as "mocking, marked by use of wit intended to cause hurt feelings." *Harsh* is a related term, and in this context the closest meaning would be "severely critical." *Genial* is a near antonym, and here it would mean "kind." *Heartfelt* means, "coming from a place of strong and sincere emotion."

20. B: An *egress* is an exit from a place. While exiting during a fire alarm, one might proceed through or to the other options which could be defined as follows: (1) *hallway*, which means, "the passage corridor," (2) *shelter*, which means, "something that offers protection from danger (or cover from weather)," and (3) outdoors, which means, "into the open air."

21. C: *Equivalence* is a synonym for *parity*, which means "the state or fact of being exactly identical in number, amount, status, or quality." Therefore, *inequality* is an antonym. *Similarity* is a related word implying presence of qualities in common. *Competition* could fit into this sentence, and in this context this word means, "the process of trying to win or do better than another."

22. B: The verbs *estrange* and *alienate* both mean "to cause someone to change from a friendly or loving attitude to one that is unfriendly or hostile." *Antagonize* is a related verb meaning to "instill bitter feelings in or make angry." *Endear* is a near antonym defined as "to make someone or something liked or loved." *Encourage* has a number of meanings, and in this sentence the closest applicable meaning would be "to give someone hope or confidence."

23. D: *Unnecessary* is a synonym for *gratuitous*, which means "not needed under the circumstances and unjustifiable." *Irrelevant* is a related term meaning, "having nothing to do with the matter at hand." Hateful means, "spitefully malicious." Excessive means, "beyond what is considered necessary".

24. B: In this sentence, *voracious* is a synonym for gluttonous, which means "very hungry." Voracious can also mean "unusually eager or enthusiastic." *Hearty* is a related term; of its numerous meanings, the closest meaning for this sentence would be "substantial." In this sentence, *minimal* means "very small." In the context of this sentence, *bland* would mean,

"lacking flavor," but the term would be more appropriate for defining the person's diet rather than their appetite.

25. A: *Laterally* is synonymous with *sideways*; both mean "to the side." All of the other choices are also directional adverbs which mean "to the front" (forward), "toward the rear" (backward), and "toward a higher level" (upward). All of these terms have other meanings as well.

26. B: *Brave* and *dauntless* both mean "feeling or showing no fear by nature." *Overconfident* is a related term that in this instance would mean "overly self-assured." Fearful is an antonym, which here would mean "afraid." *Disconsolate* is another word for "sad."

27. D: *Distrustfully* is a synonym for *askance*, which means "with distrust." *Incredulously* is a similar term meaning "showing disbelief." *Contemptuously* means, "showing or feeling strong dislike or lack of respect." *Encouragingly* essentially is synonymous with "hopefully."

28. B: *Hitherto* is an adverb signifying "thus far"; it also can mean "up to a particular time." The other listed terms refer more to quality than timing. *Properly* means "correctly or in a suitable manner." *Completely* means "fully or thoroughly." *Sufficiently* implies some subjectivity, as it is defined as "enough, to a degree or quantity that satisfies one's expectations or requirements."

29. A: *Sage* is used as adjective here and is therefore synonymous with one definition of *wise*, which is "possessing or displaying profound understanding and intelligent application of knowledge." Sage can also be a noun describing a "wise or learned individual." *Astute* is a related adjective meaning, "possessing or displaying practical shrewdness or judgment." *Vast* means "unusually large," and *logical* conveys that something is "based on facts, rational deliberation, and sensible analysis."

30. C: *Mitigate* is a synonym for the verb *help* in its sense that means, "to make more tolerable or less severe." Rectify is a related but stronger verb meaning, "to correct." Lessen as used here is synonymous with "decrease." In this sentence, *disguise* would mean would mean "to hide feelings or facts from someone."

31. A: *Forthright* and *frank* both mean "open and honest about expressing one's true opinion." *Reticent* is almost the opposite, as it means, "reserved, not willing to talk very freely." *Evasive* means, "avoiding an issue or trouble." Animated in this sentence would connote that her conversations are "full of liveliness or energy."

32. D: *Dyspeptic* has the same definition as *ill-tempered*, meaning in this case "possessing or exhibiting a habitually bad temper." Dyspeptic can also mean, "having acid indigestion". *Sullen* is a similar term that as used here signifies, "displaying hostile or resentful silence." *Erratic* has several meanings that could apply here, including "random," "fitful," and "uneven." Comatose literally can mean "in a coma," but it also can be defined as "unable to function."

33. A: *Intensity* is a synonym for vehemence, which is defined as "a state or quality of showing intense feeling or conviction." *Passion* has a number of meanings, some of which

are similar to vehemence, notably in the case of "depth of feeling or ardor (another choice)" or "intense enthusiasm." Duplicity means "deceitfulness."

34. B: *Unflappable* and *imperturbable* both mean "not easily frightened or unnerved, able to sustain composure." All of the other terms have unrelated meanings. *Unflinching* means, "showing no signs of hesitation or yielding in purpose." *Proficient* means, "possessing or displaying extraordinary skill, knowledge, or experience." *Diligent* is the same as "busy" in the sense of "occupied with often constant activity."

35. C: *Standard* has several meanings, one of which is synonymous with "benchmark," which is defined as "an example against which things of the same type are judged." *Pinnacle* is somewhat related, meaning "the highest part or point of something." While mammography is a *test,* defined as "a procedure or operation done to settle an uncertainty," *test* is not the best answer. *Method* means "the way of or procedure for doing something."

36. C: The second paragraph of the passage notes that "up to one-third of people with peanut allergies have severe reactions." Since one-third is approximately 33%, (C) is the correct choice.

37. D: The second paragraph of the passage notes that in 2008, Duke experts stated that they expect to offer treatment in five years. Five years from 2008 is 2013.

38. B: The last sentence in paragraph five lists the cuisines in which one should watch for peanuts. Italian is not listed.

39. A: The second sentence of the first paragraph states that peanut allergy is the most common cause of food-related death.

40. C: The passage implies that it is not always easy to know which foods have traces of peanuts in them and that it's important to make sure you know what you're eating. This is hard or impossible if you share someone else's food.

41. D: Paragraph two gives examples of symptoms of peanut allergies and, more specifically, examples of symptoms of anaphylaxis. A running or stuffy nose is given as a symptom of the former, but not of the latter.

42. D: The main idea of this passage is that vaccines help the immune system function properly. One of the common traps that many test-takers fall into is assuming that the first sentence of the passage will express the main idea. Although this will be true for some passages, often the author will use the first sentence to attract interest or to make an introductory, but not central, point. On this question, if you assume that the first sentence contains the main idea, you will mistakenly choose answer B. Finding the main idea of a passage requires patience and thoroughness; you cannot expect to know the main idea until you have read the entire passage. In this case, a diligent reading will show you that answer choices A, B, and C express details from the passage, but only answer choice D is a comprehensive summary of the author's message.

43. C: This passage does not state that the symptoms of disease will not emerge until the body has learned to fight the disease. The typical structure of these questions is to ask you

to identify the answer choice that contains a detail not included in the passage. This question structure makes your work a little more difficult, because it requires you to confirm that the other three details are in the passage. In this question, the details expressed in answer choices A, B, and D are all explicit in the passage. The passage never states, however, that the symptoms of disease do not emerge until the body has learned how to fight the disease-causing microbe. On the contrary, the passage implies that a person may become quite sick and even die before the body learns to effectively fight the disease.

44. B: In the third paragraph, the word *virulent* means "malicious." Sometimes the word will be one of those used in the vocabulary section of the exam; other times, the word in question will be a slightly difficult word used regularly in academic and professional circles. In some cases, you may already know the basic definition of the word. Nevertheless, you should always go back and look at the way the word is used in the passage. The exam will often include answer choices that are legitimate definitions for the given word, but which do not express how the word is used in the passage. For instance, the word *virulent* could in some circumstances mean contagious or annoying. However, since the passage is not talking about transfer of the disease and is referring to a serious illness, malicious is the more appropriate answer.

45. C: The author's primary purpose in writing this essay is to inform. The answer choices are always the same: The author's purpose is to entertain, to persuade, to inform, or to analyze. When an author is *writing to entertain*, he or she is not including a great deal of factual information; instead, the focus is on vivid language and interesting stories. *Writing to persuade* means "trying to convince the reader of something." When a writer is just trying to provide the reader with information, without any particular bias, he or she is *writing to inform*. Finally, *writing to analyze* means to consider a subject already well known to the reader. For instance, if the above passage took an objective look at the pros and cons of various approaches to fighting disease, we would say that the passage was a piece of analysis. Because the purpose of this passage is to present new information to the reader in an objective manner, however, it is clear that the author's intention is to inform.

46. B: Hunter Gatherer is not a name the passage gives for a diet.

47. B: Dairy is listed as a food that is not allowed on the diet.

48. A: The passage notes that the idea behind the diet is that we are genetically adapted to the diet of our Paleolithic forebears.

49. B: The last sentence of the passage states that some studies support the idea of positive health benefits from the diet.

50. D: The directions indicate "for relief of headaches."

51. C: In this context upset means physical disorder.

52. C: The maximum one should take is 4 in a 24-hour period. One can call a doctor after 24 hours.

53. B: In this context, persists means continues.

54. B: Since one can take 1 pill every 4 hours, the answer is 3.

55. B: Tip number 2 best answers this detail question. The tip recommends that those who drink whole milk gradually switch to fat-free milk. Since the question asks about ways to reduce saturated fat and calories, using skim milk in the place of water does not address the issue being raised.

56. A: The author uses headings to organize the passage. While the headings are bold print, such font is not used to organize the passage (i.e. notify the reader of what information is forthcoming), but rather to draw the reader's eyes to the headings.

57. C: Tip number 2 bests answers this detail question. Reduced fat milk contains 2% fat.

58. B: Statement I and Statement II are both true statements about calcium rich foods. Canned fish, including salmon with bones, is recommended as a calcium rich food. Cheese is mentioned as a lactose-free alternative within the milk group. Statement III is false. According to the passage, condensed cream soups should be made with milk, not water.

59. D: The best choice for this question is choice (D). The other options would clarify information for minor details within the passage and would provide little new information for the reader. However, food recommendations for those who do not consume milk products are listed under a separate heading, and lactose intolerance is the only reason listed. The reader can deduce that this is a main idea in the passage and the definition of "lactose intolerance" would help explain this main idea to the reader.

60. D: The author's style is to give facts and details in a bulleted list. Of the options given, you are most likely to find this style in a health textbook. A tourist guidebook would most likely make recommendations about where to eat, not what to eat. An encyclopedia would list and define individual foods. A friendly letter would have a date, salutation, and a closing.

Mathematics Review

61. C: This is a simple addition problem involving the process of carrying. Start with the ones column and add 4+7. Write down the 1 and add the 1 to the digits in the tens column: Now add 3+7+1. Write down the 1 and add the 1 to the digits in the hundreds column. Add 6+3+1 and write down 0. Add the 1 to the digits in the thousands column. Add 4+7+1 and write down the 1. Add the 1 to the digits in the ten-thousands column. Add 1+1 and write down 2 to get the answer 21,011.

62. D: This is a simple subtraction problem. Start with the ones column and subtract 5-2, then 4-3, then 6-1, then 9-6 to get 3,513.

63. C: $29 + r = 420$
$29 + r - 29 = 420 - 29$
$r = 391$

64. D: This is a multiplication problem with carrying. Start with the ones column. Multiply 4 by each digit in above it beginning with the ones column. Write down each product: going across it will read 3572. Now multiply 6 by each of the digits above it. Write down each product: going across it will read 5358. Ensure that the 8 is in the tens column and the other numbers fall evenly to the right. Now add the numbers like a regular addition problem to get 57,152

65. C: This is a simple multiplication problem with carrying. Start with the 7 and multiply each digit above: 7 x 9 = 63. Write down the 3 and place the 6 on top of the 6. Multiply 7 x 4 to get 28. Add in the 6 to get 34. Write down the 4 and place the 3 on top of the 6. Multiply 7 x 6 to get 42. Add in the 3 to get 45. The product is 4543.

66. D: Area = length x width
$A = 7 \times 5$
$A = 35$

67. C: This is a simple division problem. Divide the 9 into 86. It goes in 9 times. Write 9 above the 6. Subtract 81 from 86 and get 5. Bring down the 3. Divide 9 into 53. It goes in 5 times. Write 4 next to the 9 and subtract 45 from 53. There is 8 remaining.

68. A: This is a simple division problem. Divide 97 into 292. It goes in 3 times. Write 3 above the second 2 and subtract 291 from 292. The result is 1. Bring down the 9. Since 19 cannot be divided into 97, write a zero next to the 3. Bring down the 4. Drive 97 into 194. It goes 2 times.

69. C: To solve, find the sum. 35% + 4% = 39%

70. D: This is multiplication with decimals. Multiply the 7 by 8 to get 56. Put down the 6 and carry the 5. Multiply 7 by 2 to get 14. Add the 5. Write 19 to left of 6. Multiply the 1 by the 8 to get 8. Multiply 1 by 2 to get 2. Add the two lines together, making sure that the 8 in the

- 79 -

bottom figure is even with the 9. Get 476. Count 4 decimal points over (2 from the top multiplier and 2 from the second multiplier) and add a 0 before adding the decimal.

71. D: To solve, divide 1.6 into .8. Move the decimal in 16 over 1 place to make it 16. Because this decimal point was moved 1 places, it must be done to the other decimal too. .8 becomes 8. Now divide 16 into 8 (not 8 into 16).

72. C: Solve as follows:
$5/8 = x/100$
$5 \cdot 100 \div 8 = x$
$x = 62.5$

73. D: Circle the 6 in the hundredths place, Look at the digit in the thousandths place. Since it is over 5, the 6 becomes 7.

74. A: Write 512 then add the decimal in the thousandths place, the third place from the right.

75. A: To solve, you will need to move the decimal 4 places. Since the scientific notation had a negative power of 10, move the decimal left. If the power of 10 had been positive, you would have needed to move it to the right. In this problem, solve as follows:
7.4×10^{-4}
$7.4 \times 1/10,000$
7.4×0.0001
0.00074

76. A: To divide fractions, change the second fraction to its reciprocal (its reverse) and multiply: $3/5 \times 2/1$

77. A: To solve, test each answer. Notice the in (A), the numerator has been multiplied by 3 to get 12. The denominator has been multiplied by 3 to get 21. In (B) the numerator has been multiplied by 4 and the denominator has been multiplied by 5. In (C), the numerator has been multiplied by 3 and the denominator has been multiplied by 4. In (D), the numerator has been multiplied by 4 and the denominator has been multiplied by a number less than 4.

78. D: The denominator has been multiplied by 3 to get 21. Think of what number multiplied by 3 totals 18.

79. B: Add to solve. The height of the window from the floor is not needed in this equation. It is extra information. You only need to add the heights of the two bookcases. Change the fractions so that they have a common denominator. After you add, simplify the fraction.
$14\frac{1}{2} + 8\frac{3}{4}$
$= 14\ 2/4 + 8\frac{3}{4}$
$= 22\ 5/4$
$= 23\frac{1}{4}$

80. A: Divide 68 by 7. The answer is 9 with a remainder of 5.

81. A: Divide 3 by 60 to get .05 or 5%

82. D: Divide 1 by 25 to get .04 or 4%.

83. B: $y = x + 5$, and you were told that $x = -3$. Fill in the missing information for x, then solve.
$y = (-3) + 5$
$y = 2$

84. D: To solve, first get both fractions on the same side of the equation to isolate the percentage sign. When 5/6 is moved to the opposite side of the equation, it must be divided by the fraction there: $1/3 \div 5/6$.

To divide one fraction into another, multiply by the reciprocal of the denominator: $1/3 \times 6/5 = 6/15 = 2/5 = 40\%$.

85. D: To change a fraction to a decimal, divide the numerator (5.00) by the denominator (8).

86. B: To change a decimal to a percent, multiply it by 100 by moving the decimal point two spaces to the right.

87. C: Let x stand for the amount that it would cost to make the 12-minute call. Solve with the following equation:
$15/2.50 = 12/x$
Cross multiply, as follows:
$15 \cdot x = 2.50 \cdot 12$
$15x = 30.00$
Divide each side by 15.
$15x/15 = 30.00/15$
$x = \$2.00$

88. D: To solve, rewrite the equation with a decimal in place of the percent:
$12 = .25x$
$x = 12/.25 = 1200/25 = 48$

89. D: To solve, change the percent to a decimal:
$.32x = 96$
$x = 96/.32 = 9600/32 = 300$

90. B: Since they are like terms, just subtract. The result will be a negative number.

91. D: Think of the numbers as they would appear on a number line to place them in the correct order.

92. B: To solve, first do the operations in parenthesis, then add like terms:
$4x + 8 - 12 + 3x + 15 = 7x + 20$

93. D: To solve, get like terms on opposite sides of the equation: $4x = 28$; $x = 7$

94. B: To solve, first do the operations in parenthesis, then add/subtract like terms in order to get like terms on opposite sides of the equation: $2r + 8 + 8 = 4r + 12$
$2r + 16 = 4r + 12$; $4 = 2r$; $r = 2$

95. C: In this problem, if you do not know how to solve, try filling in the answer choices to see which one checks out. Many math problems may be solved by a guess and check method when you have a selection of answer choices.
$27 - x = -5$
$x = 32$

96. D: -10 is greater than -(-(-15)), which can also be written as -15.

97. A: Volume = LWH. Here that is 14 x 10 x 3 = 420.

98. B: $2^3 + (4 + 1) = 2 \times 2 \times 2 + 5 = 8 + 5 = 13$.

99. B: (4 x 9) – (1/2 x 6) = 36 – 3 = 33.

100. A: The correct answer is B = 3A - 2.

Science Review

101. B: The adrenal glands are part of the endocrine system. They sit on the kidneys and produce hormones that regulate salt and water balance and influence blood pressure and heart rate.

102. C: An ionic bond forms when one atom donates an electron from its outer shell, called a valence electron, to another atom to form two oppositely charged atoms.

103. B: Metals are usually solids at room temperature, while nonmetals are usually gases at room temperature.

104. D: A solution that contains more hydroxide ions than hydrogen ions is a base, and bases have a pH greater than 7, so the only possible answer is D, 9.

105. B: Magnesium oxide cannot be found on the periodic table because it is a compound of two elements.

106. C: Potential energy is stored energy. At the top of the hill, the cyclist has the greatest amount of potential energy (and the least amount of kinetic energy) because his motion is decreased and he has the potential of motion in any direction.

107. A: The trait Ll describes the genotype of the person or the traits for the genes they carry. It is heterozygous because it contains a dominant gene and a recessive gene. Tallness is the phenotype of the person or the physical expression of the genes they carry, because L for tallness is the dominant gene.

108. B: Coulomb's law describes the electric force between two charged particles. It states that like charges repel and opposite charges attract, and the greater their distance, the less force they will exert on each other.

109. C: *Ribosomes* are the organelles that organize protein synthesis. A ribosome, composed of RNA and protein, is a tiny structure responsible for putting proteins together. The *mitochondrion* converts chemical energy into a form that is more useful for the functions of the cell. The *nucleus* is the central structure of the cell. It contains the DNA and administrates the functions of the cell. The *vacuole* is a cell organelle in which useful materials (for example, carbohydrates, salts, water, and proteins) are stored.

110. D: The mass of 1.0 mol oxygen gas is 32 grams. The molar mass of oxygen can be obtained from the periodic table. In most versions of the table, the molar mass of the element is directly beneath the full name of the element. There is a little trick to this question. Oxygen is a diatomic molecule, which means that it always appears in pairs. In order to determine the mass in grams of 1.0 mol of oxygen gas, then, you must double the molar mass. The listed mass is 16, so the correct answer to the problem is 32.

111. A: An adult inhales 500 mL of air in an average breath. Interestingly, humans can inhale about eight times as much air in a single breath as they do in an average breath. People tend to take a larger breath after making a larger inhalation. This is one reason that many breathing therapies, for instance those incorporated into yoga practice, focus on making a complete exhalation. The process of respiration is managed by the autonomic nervous system. The body requires a constant replenishing of oxygen, so even brief interruptions in respiration can be damaging or fatal.

112. D: During *meiosis I*, the chromosome number is reduced from diploid to haploid. *Interphase* is the period of the cell cycle that occurs in between divisions of the cell. In *meiosis*, the homologous chromosomes in a diploid cell separate, reducing the number of chromosomes in each cell by half. *Mitosis* is the phase of cell division in which the cell nucleus divides. *S phase* is the part of the mitotic cycle in which DNA is synthesized.

113. D: Gamma radiation has no charge. This form of electromagnetic radiation can travel a long distance and can penetrate the human body. Sunlight and radio waves are both examples of gamma radiation. Alpha radiation has a 2+ charge. It only travels short distances and cannot penetrate clothing or skin. Radium and uranium both emit alpha radiation. Beta radiation has a 1– charge. It can travel several feet through the air and is capable of penetrating the skin. This kind of radiation can be damaging to health over a long period of exposure. There is no such thing as delta radiation.

114. D: The force of *blood pressure* motivates filtration in the kidneys. *Filtration* is the process through which the kidneys remove waste products from the body. All of the water in the blood passes through the kidneys every 45 minutes. Waste products are diverted into ducts and excreted from the body, while the healthy components of the water in blood are reabsorbed into the bloodstream. *Peristalsis* is the set of involuntary muscle movements that move food through the digestive system.

115. A: Liquid is the densest form of water. Water can exist in three states, depending on temperature. Ranging from coldest to hottest, these states are solid, liquid, and gaseous—or ice, water, and steam. Water freezes at zero degrees Celsius. Although the solidity of ice might lead one to believe that it is the densest form of water, water actually expands about nine percent when it is frozen. This is the reason why ice will float in water. Steam is the least dense form of water.

116. A: When forward and reverse chemical reactions are taking place at the same rate, a chemical reaction has achieved equilibrium. This means that the respective concentrations of reactants and products do not change over time. In theory, a chemical reaction will remain in equilibrium indefinitely. One of the common tasks in the chemistry lab is to find the equilibrium constant (or set of relative concentrations that result in equilibrium) for a given reaction. In thermal equilibrium, there is no net heat exchange between a body and its surroundings. In dynamic equilibrium, any motion in one direction is offset by an equal motion in the other direction.

117. A: *Insulin* decreases the concentration of blood glucose. It is produced by the pancreas. *Glucagon* is a hormone produced by the pancreas. Glucagon acts in opposition to insulin, motivating an increase in the levels of blood sugar. *Growth hormone* is secreted by the pituitary gland. It is responsible for the growth of the body, specifically by metabolizing

proteins, carbohydrates, and lipids. The *glucocorticoids* are a group of steroid hormones that are produced by the adrenal cortex. The glucocorticoids contribute to the metabolism of carbohydrates, proteins, and fats.

118. B: *Interphase* is the longest phase in the life of a cell. Interphase occurs between cell divisions. *Prophase* is the initial stage of mitosis. It is also the longest stage. During prophase, the chromosomes become visible, and the centrioles divide and position themselves on either side of the nucleus. *Anaphase* is the third phase of mitosis, in which chromosome pairs divide and take up positions on opposing poles. *Metaphase* is the second stage of mitosis. In it, the chromosomes align themselves across the center of the cell.

119. B: 119°K is equivalent to –154 degrees Celsius. To convert degrees Kelvin to degrees Celsius, simply subtract 273. To convert degrees Celsius to degrees Kelvin, simply add 273. To convert degrees Kelvin into degrees Fahrenheit, multiply by 9/5 and subtract 460. To convert degrees Fahrenheit to degrees Kelvin, add 460 and then multiply by 5/9. To convert degrees Celsius to degrees Fahrenheit, multiply by 9/5 and then add 32. To convert degrees Fahrenheit to degrees Celsius, subtract 32 and then multiply by 5/9.

120. C: Forty percent of female blood volume is composed of red blood cells. Red blood cells, otherwise known as erythrocytes, are large and do not have a nucleus. These cells are produced in the bone marrow and carry oxygen throughout the body. White blood cells, also known as leukocytes, make up about 1% of the blood volume. About 55% of the blood volume is made up of plasma, which itself is primarily composed of water. The plasma in blood supplies cells with nutrients and removes metabolic waste. Blood also contains platelets, otherwise known as thrombocytes, which are essential to effective blood clotting.

121. A: Bacterial cells do not contain *mitochondria*. Bacteria are prokaryotes composed of single cells; their cell walls contain peptidoglycans. The functions normally performed in the mitochondria are performed in the cell membrane of the bacterial cell. *DNA* is the nucleic acid that contains the genetic information of the organism. It is in the shape of a double helix. DNA can reproduce itself and can synthesize RNA. A *vesicle* is a small cavity containing fluid. A *ribosome* is a tiny particle composed of RNA and protein, in which polypeptides are constructed.

122. B: The *joule* is the SI unit of energy. Energy is the ability to do work or generate heat. In regard to electrical energy, a joule is the amount of electrical energy required to pass a current of one ampere through a resistance of one ohm for one second. In physical or mechanical terms, the joule is the amount of energy required for a force of one newton to act over a distance of one meter. The *ohm* is a unit of electrical resistance. The *henry* is a unit of inductance. The *newton* is a unit of force.

123. B: High-density lipoproteins (*HDL*) are considered to be the healthiest form of cholesterol. This type of cholesterol actually reduces the risk of heart disease. A lipoprotein is composed of both lipid and protein. These substances cannot move through the bloodstream by themselves; they must be carried along by some other substance. Although most people think of cholesterol as an unhealthy substance, it helps to maintain cell walls and produce hormones. Cholesterol is also important in the production of vitamin D and the bile acids that aid digestion. The other answer choices are low-density lipoproteins (*LDL*), very-low-density lipoproteins (*VLDL*), and very-high-density lipoproteins (*VHDL*).

124. D: Deoxyribonucleic acid (*DNA*) is not involved in translation. *Translation* is the process by which messenger RNA (*mRNA*) messages are decoded into polypeptide chains. Transfer RNA (*tRNA*) is a molecule that moves amino acids into the ribosomes during the synthesis of protein. Messenger RNA carries sets of instructions for the conversion of amino acids into proteins from the RNA to the other parts of the cell. *Ribosomes* are the tiny particles in the cell where proteins are put together. Ribosomes are composed of ribonucleic acid (RNA) and protein.

125. A: A *mass spectrometer* separates gaseous ions according to their mass-to-charge ratio. This machine is used to distinguish the various elements in a piece of matter. An *interferometer* measures the wavelength of light by comparing the interference phenomena of two waves: an experimental wave and a reference wave. A *magnetometer* measures the direction and magnitude of a magnetic field. Finally, a *capacitance meter* measures the capacitance of a capacitor. Some sophisticated capacitance meters may also measure inductance, leakage, and equivalent series resistance.

126. A: Gas exchange occurs in the *alveoli*, the minute air sacs on the interior of the lungs. The *bronchi* are large cartilage-based tubes of air; they extend from the end of the trachea into the lungs, where they branch apart. The *larynx*, which houses the vocal cords, is positioned between the trachea and the pharynx; it is involved in swallowing, breathing, and speaking. The *pharynx* extends from the nose to the uppermost portions of the trachea and esophagus. In order to enter these two structures, air and other matter must pass through the pharynx.

127. C: There are four different nucleotides in DNA. *Nucleotides* are monomers of nucleic acids, composed of five-carbon sugars, a phosphate group, and a nitrogenous base. Nucleotides make up both DNA and RNA. They are essential for the recording of an organism's genetic information, which guides the actions of the various cells of the body. Nucleotides are also a crucial component of adenosine triphosphate (ATP), one of the parts of DNA and a chemical that enables metabolism and muscle contractions.

128. A: Van der Waals forces are the weak forces of attraction between two molecules. The van der Waals force is considered to be any of the attractive or repulsive forces between electrons that are not related to electrostatic interaction or covalent bonds. Compared to other chemical bonds, the strength of van der Waals forces is small. However, these forces have a great effect on a substance's solubility and other characteristics.

129. B: In the lungs, oxygen is transported from the air to the blood through the process of *diffusion*. Specifically, the alveolar membranes withdraw the oxygen from the air in the lungs into the bloodstream. *Osmosis* is the movement of a solution from an area of low concentration to an area of higher concentration through a permeable membrane. *Dissipation* is any wasteful consumption or use. *Reverse osmosis* is a process for purifying a solution by forcing it through a membrane that blocks only certain pollutants.

130. D: The *electron transport system* enacted during aerobic respiration requires oxygen. This is the last component of biological oxidation. *Osmosis* is the movement of fluid from an area of high concentration through a partially permeable membrane to an area of lower concentration. This process usually stops when the concentration is the same on either side

of the membrane. *Glycolysis* is the initial step in the release of glucose energy. The *Krebs cycle* is the last phase of the process in which cells convert food into energy. It is during this stage that carbon dioxide is produced and hydrogen is extracted from molecules of carbon.

131. C: The correct formula for converting Fahrenheit measurements to Celsius measurements is 5/9 (F+32), where F=temperature in Fahrenheit.

132. A: A calorimeter is used to measure changes in heat. This instrument uses a thermometer to measure the amount of energy necessary to increase the temperature of water.

133. C: Vectors have a magnitude (e.g., 5 meters/second) and direction (e.g., towards north). Of the choice listed, only velocity has a direction. (35 m/s north, for example). Speed, distance and time are all quantities that have a size but not a direction. That's why, for example, a car's speedometer reads 35 miles/hour, but does not indicate your direction of travel.

134. A: According to the Dana system, minerals that contain the anion SO_4^{2-} are part of the sulfate class. Sulfate minerals are typically formed in environments where highly saline water evaporates. Gypsum is an example of a mineral that belongs to the sulfate class.

135. B: The total energy of an isolated system is always conserved. However the mechanical energy may not be, since some mechanical energy could be converted into radiation (light) or heat (through friction). According to Einstein's famous equation $E = mc^2$, energy is (occasionally, like in nuclear reactions!) converted into mass, and vice versa, where c is the speed of light. This does not affect the conservation of energy law, however, since the mass is considered to have an energy equivalent. This equation does not tell anything about the mechanical energy of a particle; it just shows how much energy would be generated if the mass was converted directly into energy.

136. C: Physical weathering of rocks can be caused by changes in temperature and pressure, as well as the freezing and thawing of water on the surfaces of rocks. Oxidation is a chemical process, not a physical one. Therefore, it is considered an example of chemical rather than physical weathering.

137. B: Medical ultrasound machines use echolocation, in which sound waves are bounced off objects and the returning sound waves are used to create an image. This same process is also used by some animals, such as bats and dolphins. The spectrum of sound has three areas: infrasonic, audible, and ultrasonic. Humans can hear sound waves between 20 Hz and 20,000 Hz, so these are the cut-off points. The Doppler effect refers to the changing pitch of sound for objects that are moving towards or away from you.

138. B: A closed thermodynamic system can exchange heat and work, but not matter, with its surrounding environment. In contrast, an isolated system cannot exchange heat, work, or matter with its surrounding environment, so its mass and energy levels always remain constant. Open systems can exchange heat, work, and mass with their surrounding environments.

139. B: If the charged object is negative, it will cause electrons in the neutral object to move away from the charged object. If the charged object is positive, it will attract electrons. In both cases, there will be an attractive force. There is also an induced repulsive force, but the repulsive force is less because the like charges are farther away. An object has a net charge because electrons have been added to a neutral object or electrons have been removed from the atoms, ions, or molecules in the object.

140. B: Answer B correctly states the definition of a conductor. Answer C is incorrect because a current will also flow in an insulator, for example, although that current will be very low. In metals, the current flow caused by an electric field is much greater than in an insulator or semiconductor because the electrons are not bound to any particular atom, but are free to move. Answer D is incorrect because a vacuum tube is a device that electrons can flow in, butut a vacuum tube is not considered a conductor.

141. A: Quartzite, marble, and slate are all examples of metamorphic rocks, while granite is one of the most common types of igneous rocks.

142. A: In a Zn-Cu battery, the zinc terminal has a higher concentration of electrons than the copper terminal, so there is a potential difference between the locations of the two terminals. This is a form of electrical energy brought about by the chemical interactions between the metals and the electrolyte the battery uses. Creating a circuit and causing a current to flow will transform the electrical energy into heat energy, mechanical energy, or another form of electrical energy, depending on the devices in the circuit. A generator transforms mechanical energy into electrical energy and a transformer changes the electrical properties of a form of electrical energy.

143. C: A ray of sunlight consists of many different colors of light. The speed of red light in water is slightly larger than the speed of violet light, so the angle of refraction of violet light is greater than that of red light. This causes the light to separate and creates a spectrum of colors, like in a prism. Raindrops do exhibit total internal reflection for all the wavelengths inside the droplet, although this is not what causes the rainbow. Instead, this causes a second refraction as the sunlight emerges from the water droplet, which can sometimes been seen in nature as a "double rainbow."

144. C: The state of matter in which atoms have the strongest bond is the solid state. Matter, which is defined as any substance that has mass and occupies space, can exist as a solid, liquid, gas, or plasma. The atoms or molecules that form solids possess the strongest bonds, while those that form plasma possess the weakest bonds.

145. C: Protons and neutrons are both considered nucleons. The number of nucleons in a nucleus is called the *mass number*. Isotopes of the same element have different mass numbers. But since they are the same element, they must have the same atomic number, which is equal to the number of protons. Thus, only the number of neutrons changes, since electron's mass is so low that it doesn't have much effect on the mass number of an element. Unless they are also ionized, they would have the same number of protons and electrons.

146. A: The kinetic energy of the gas molecules is directly proportional to the temperature. If the temperature decreases, so does the molecular motion. A decrease in temperature will

not necessarily mean a gas condenses to a liquid. Neither the mass nor the density is impacted, as no material was added or removed, and the volume remained the same.

147. A: Chemical compounds are formed when valence electrons from atoms of two different elements are shared or transferred. Valence electrons are the electrons located in the outermost shell of the atom, and they occupy the highest energy level. Atoms may form compounds by sharing valence electrons (covalent bonding) or by transferring electrons.

148. C: To add and subtract vectors algebraically, you add and subtract their components. To add vectors graphically, you shift the location of the vectors so that they are connected tail-to-tail. The resultant is a vector that starts at the tail of the first vector and ends at the tip of the second. To subtract vectors, however, you connect the vectors tail-to-tail, not tip to tail, starting with the vector that is not subtracted, and ending with the one that is. Think of this just like vector addition, except the vector that is subtracted (the one with the negative sign in front of it) switches directions.

149. B: The process that causes lithospheric plates to move over the surface of the mantle is called convection. The liquid in the lower portion of the mantle is heated by the Earth's core and rises to the surface, pushing aside cooler liquid that is already there. This liquid cools, and is in turn pushed aside by hotter liquid that has risen from below. This cycle, called convection, creates constant movement in the mantle that contributes to the motion of the tectonic plates.

150. A: Nuclear reactions convert mass into energy ($E = mc^2$). The mass of products is always less than that of the starting materials since some mass is now energy.

151. C: Catalysts lower the energy barrier between products and reactants and thus increase the reaction rate.

152. C: Proteins are large polypeptides, comprised of many amino acids linked together by an amide bond. DNA and RNA are made up of nucleic acids. Carbohydrates are long chains of sugars. Triglycerides are fats and are composed of a glycerol molecule and three fatty acids.

153. D: Galena, pyrite, and magnetite are examples of minerals with a metallic luster. Opal is an example of a mineral with a greasy luster, and diamonds have an adamantine luster. Muscovite and stilbite are examples of minerals with a pearly luster. Other types of luster include dull, silky, waxy, and sub-metallic.

154. C: The closer the data points are to each other, the more precise the data. This does not mean the data is accurate, but that the results are very reproducible.

155. A: Density is mass per volume, typically expressed in units such as g/cm^3, or kg/m^3.

156. B: The fact that water's specific heat capacity is second only to that of ammonia means that it takes more energy to increase the temperature of ammonia than it does to increase the temperature of water. Specific heat capacity refers to the amount of energy required to increase the temperature of a substance by one degree Celsius. Ammonia has the highest specific heat capacity of all substances, and the specific heat capacity of water is the second

highest.

157. D: Electrons are elementary particles with no known components, so it is not true that they have a nucleus. Electrons are negatively charged, and they are arranged in levels. Electrons gravitate toward the lowest energy level possible, and they have very little mass (roughly 1/1836 of the mass of a proton).

158. A: Communities around the world who drink fluoridated water have shown dramatic decreases in the number of dental cavities formed per citizen versus those communities that do not drink fluoridated water.

159. C: In geochronology, an eon is the longest time period, lasting at least half a billion years. An era lasts several hundred million years, an epoch measures tens of millions of years, and an age is shorter than 10 million years but longer than one million years.

160. C: The atomic number of an element is defined by the total number of protons it contains, and elements are arranged on the periodic table by atomic number. The atomic mass of an element is the sum total of its protons and electrons.